AHRQ Annual Report on Research and Financial Management, FY 2001

www.ahrq.gov

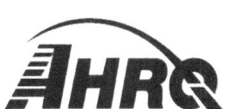

Department of Health and Human Services
Agency for Healthcare Research and Quality
February 2002
AHRQ Publication No. 02-0008

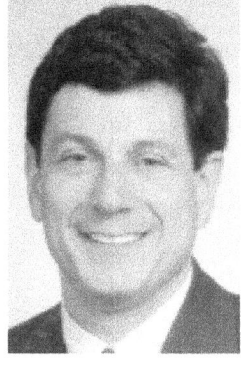

Message from the Director

I am pleased to present the Agency for Healthcare Research and Quality's FY 2001 Accountability Report, which conveys the Agency's key program and financial management activities and highlights what we have accomplished with the resources entrusted to us.

This report demonstrates how the research sponsored by AHRQ provides the scientific foundation for the Nation's efforts to improve the quality, safety, and cost-effectiveness of health care, as well as developing strategies to broaden access to services. The Agency supports the work of health services researchers at the Nation's leading academic centers through extramural grants and contracts and maintains a rigorous intramural research program that collects and analyzes data to understand changes in health care quality, cost, use, and access. AHRQ also supports efforts to develop the tools and information used by the public and private sectors to measure and improve health care quality.

FY 2001 was a very dynamic year for AHRQ. We completed a seamless transition to our new identity as the Agency for Healthcare Research and Quality. As we have affirmed over the last year, the new name is more than symbolic. As AHRQ, we have cemented our role as the lead Federal agency supporting and conducting research to improve quality, enhance the outcomes and effectiveness of health care services, and identify strategies to improve access, foster appropriate use, and reduce unnecessary expenditures.

Our research portfolio, which reflects the needs of our customers, is making a difference in the health of the public. Through our Translating Research into Practice (TRIP) program, the findings of our research conducted by AHRQ staff and grantees are being translated into improvements in clinical care and in the structure and delivery of health care services. As part of that agenda, we are making a concerted effort to track the impact of our research.

Over the last year, we have supported new investigator-initiated projects from the best and brightest health services researchers, and we have funded new targeted initiatives to help ensure that Americans get high-quality, safe health care. Among the new initiatives is a $50 million program in patient safety research—the largest single investment of its kind in this critical research area by the Federal Government. We also supported training programs that have helped nurture the careers of established health services researchers and given a boost to new investigators.

AHRQ also has continued to work in partnership with our fellow Federal agencies and with private-sector organizations to improve the quality and safety of health care services, For example, in FY 2001, AHRQ in partnership with the Centers for Disease Control and Prevention, the Food and Drug Administration, and the Centers for Medicare & Medicaid Services, established the Patient Safety Task Force to improve existing systems to collect data on patient safety. The goal of this Task Force is to identify the data that health care providers, States, and others need to collect in order to improve patient safety.

Our long-standing programs continue to inform health care decisions made at all levels of the health care system, while our newer programs are releasing findings that promise to have a significant impact on the health care system. Also, the third U.S. Preventive Services Task Force has begun to release recommendations that will greatly enhance the preventive services patients receive.

Looking ahead, I am confident that our future will be very bright and that we will have many more accomplishments to celebrate. The end result of our research will be measurable improvements in health care in America, gauged in terms of improved quality of life and patient outcomes, lives saved, and value gained for what we spend. I am proud of our accomplishments to date and look forward to building on our past successes to achieve new gains for the American people.

John M. Eisenberg, M.D.
Director
Agency for Healthcare Research and Quality

John M. Eisenberg, M.D.
1946 - 2002

This report is dedicated to the memory of AHRQ director John M. Eisenberg, M.D. Dr. Eisenberg passed away on March 10, 2002, following a year-long illness, just as this report was going to press. He had been director of AHRQ since 1997. All of his colleagues at AHRQ and in the Department of Health and Human Services mourn his untimely passing.

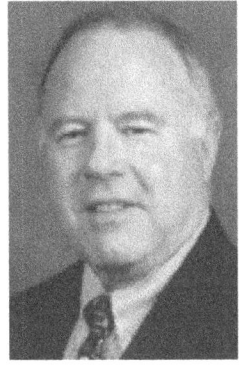

Message from the Chief Financial Officer (CFO)

I take pride in the organizational, systems, and financial accountability improvements AHRQ achieved in FY 2001. In this report, we address our efforts to link our budget, program, and financial performance information; highlight major programmatic and managerial accomplishments; and interpret and analyze our financial performance.

We are continuing to strengthen AHRQ's business practices to ensure that Agency resources are used appropriately, efficiently, and effectively. These efforts include the use of new and existing technologies and strategies, such as electronic mail or messaging, the World Wide Web, electronic bulletin boards, purchase cards, electronic funds transfer, and electronic data interchange. We also are taking steps to enhance management of AHRQ's information systems infrastructure, with a focus on information security that directly maps to the Department's Information Technology 5-Year Strategic Plan.

We reorganized and revised AHRQ's performance plan to enhance its clarity and usefulness as a strategic management tool. The revised plan is more closely aligned with goals that reflect the agency's vision, mission, and strategic goals. As a result of the increased emphasis on strategic planning, evaluation activities have assumed a greater role in overall Agency operations. Evaluations are used to demonstrate the impact of Agency work on the health care system, test and improve the usefulness and usability of agency products, and assess the effectiveness and efficiencies of internal operations. The results of the evaluation studies are used to make planning, budget, and operations decisions in subsequent years.

In response to AHRQ's expanding scope and mission, we completed four workforce planning related activities this year: evaluating the Agency's recruitment process, more clearly defining work functions and processes, refining the technical competencies needed by staff, and developing a comprehensive 5-year workforce restructuring plan that reflects Agency needs and departmental priorities. A number of followup activities are planned in FY 2002.

As acting CFO, my goals are to promote sound financial management through effective leadership, insightful policy development, and unobtrusive oversight; create an infrastructure to carry out financial management policies; and produce timely and reliable financial information about our programs. I believe this report demonstrates the strides AHRQ has made as we continue to work toward these goals.

Barry Flaer
Acting Chief Financial Officer

v

Contents

AHRQ Activities and Accomplishments, FY2001

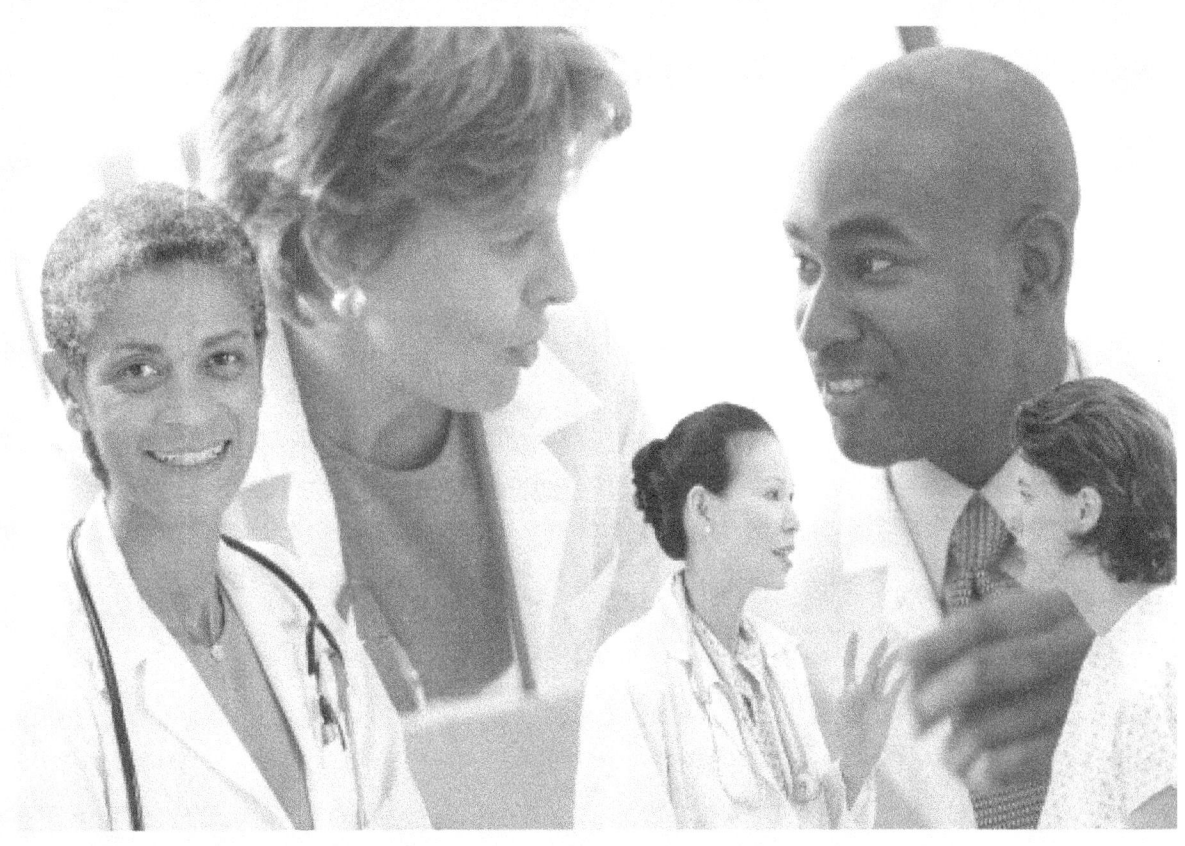

AHRQ and Health Care Today

In the first decade of the 21st century, the Nation faces critical challenges in health care. A combination of unprecedented advances in health care treatments and rapidly increasing health care costs requires the use of scientific evidence to assure that those most likely to benefit receive effective services and that the return on our investment in health care results in improved health.

Research on these and other pressing issues is at the center of the mission of the Agency for Healthcare Research and Quality. Our goal at AHRQ is to support and conduct research that addresses and anticipates health care challenges facing policymakers, health system leaders, clinicians, patients, and families. These challenges include quality of care, patient safety, access to effective care, and the costs of care.

The first section of this report presents information on the programs and activities undertaken by AHRQ in FY 2001 and provides examples of some recent accomplishments. The second section of the report presents financial statements and detailed information about AHRQ's resources and expenditures.

To set the stage for this discussion, this report presents information about the state of health care in America today and describes the role AHRQ can play in addressing some of the most important challenges and questions facing the Nation's health care system in these first few years of a new century. The report also presents AHRQ's organizational structure and key responsibilities of functional components, describes the Agency's National Advisory Council, and identifies the various audiences and customers who use the findings from Agency-supported research.

Addressing Health Care Challenges

Today, we are looking for answers to deal with escalating health care costs, a vulnerable population of uninsured Americans, continuing difficulties with access to care for some people, and disparities in care and outcomes, related not only to insurance but also to race, sex, age, health status, and geographic location.

Findings from AHRQ's Medical Expenditure Panel Survey (MEPS) and Healthcare Cost and Utilization Project (HCUP), as well as other sources, provide a snapshot of health care in America today. For example:

Health Care Costs

- Approximately 84 percent of the U.S community population has at least some medical expenses during a year. In 1998, the average expense per person for those individuals was just over $2,400.

- Overall, most expenses for the community population are covered by private insurance. In 1998, for example, about 39 percent of all expenditures for people living in the community were paid by private insurance.

- Approximately one-fifth of expenses for the community population are paid out-of-pocket. In 1998, for example, about 19 percent of all expenditures for this population were paid out-of-pocket, 24 percent were paid by Medicare, and 9 percent were paid by Medicaid.

- In 1998, only 56 percent of the uninsured community population had any medical expenses, compared with 87 percent for those with private insurance. Medical expenditures for the uninsured also are substantially lower than for the insured and are largely, but not exclusively, paid out-of-pocket.

- The distribution of medical expenditures is highly skewed: 1 percent of the population accounts for more than 25 percent of all expenses, and 5 percent of the population accounts for more than half of the total.

Health Insurance

- Today, about 16 percent of Americans are uninsured.

- More than 33 percent of young adults aged 19 to 24 are uninsured.

- As of 2000, about 3.3 million uninsured children were enrolled in the State Children's Health Insurance Program (SCHIP).

Resource Use

- Each year, three of every four Americans receive outpatient care from a medical provider.

- About 7 percent of the U.S. population has at least one hospital stay during the year. In 1998, about 5 percent of children birth to age 4 had a hospital stay.

- In 1998, about one in five U.S. children from birth to age 4 did not have an office-based doctor's visit.

- Health care use estimates are highest for elderly people, people in poor health, and those who die during a year.

Access to Care

- Nearly 18 percent of the population has no usual source of care.

- Hispanic Americans and young adults are more likely than others to be without a usual source of care.

- Almost 12 percent of families have members who experience difficulty or delay in obtaining health care or do not receive needed care.

- Declines in health insurance coverage are responsible for only one-fifth of the declines in access to care, meaning that increasing health insurance coverage alone will not be enough to eliminate problems in accessing care.

Health Care Disparities

- Women are less likely than white men to be referred for kidney transplants.

- Blacks are much less likely than whites to receive therapeutic procedures for several common cancers such as cancer of the colon, bladder, cervix, and breast.

- Minorities are more likely than whites to say their health status is "fair." Nearly 17 percent of Hispanic women and more than 15 percent of black women say they are in fair or poor health, compared with 11 percent of white women.

- Women of color have higher rates of high blood pressure, tend to develop it at an earlier age, and are less likely than white women to receive treatment for it.

- Minority women, particularly black women, are at relatively high risk for giving birth to low birthweight infants, both prematurely and at term. Maternal and infant deaths among black women are 5 and 2.5 times greater, respectively, than the national average.

- Black women have a higher incidence of fibroids, larger and more numerous fibroids when first diagnosed, and a higher rate of hysterectomies than women of other races. Yet black women are more likely than white or Hispanic women to have their fibroids surgically removed through a myomectomy, a procedure that preserves the uterus.

Role and Mission of the Agency for Healthcare Research and Quality

The Agency for Healthcare Research and Quality is recognized as the Federal agency uniquely positioned to address the health care challenges we face today. The health services research supported and conducted by AHRQ is different from but

AHRQ at a Glance

Budget: $270 million in FY 2001

Staff: 292

Director: John M. Eisenberg, M.D., M.B.A.

Deputy Director: Lisa Simpson, M.B., B.Ch., M.P.H.

complementary to the research performed in laboratories. The data gathered for AHRQ-funded health services research comes from:

- People receiving the care and the clinicians and systems providing the care.

- Employees enrolled in health plans (to help measure and improve patients' experiences with care).

- Hospital records and administrative data provided by States working together to obtain detailed information about the health care people receive.

- Clinicians who meticulously examine and evaluate hundreds of research articles to synthesize the information for clinicians and patients. The results enhance access to relevant evidence for making effective clinical decisions.

Health services research completes the work begun in the laboratory. Health services researchers strive to answer the central question: "Does this work in daily practice with real people whose characteristics, needs, and local communities are different?"

Rapid changes in the financing and organization of health care, changing characteristics and health care needs of the U.S. population, and the proliferation of new health care services make the need for high-quality health services research more critical than ever. The future of the field and the vision for health services research come from the scientific community—investigators who are on the front lines of the clinical, health system, and health policy problems that are waiting to be resolved through health services research. The nurturing of novel research approaches, concepts, and directions is central to AHRQ's mission, and it is essential to providing effective health care in the Nation.

AHRQ supports and conducts health services research on:

- Outcomes
- Quality of Care
- Patient safety

- Costs of care
- Use of services
- Access to Care

4

The mission of the Agency for Healthcare Research and Quality is to support, conduct, and disseminate research that improves the outcomes, quality, access to, cost, and use of health care services and enhance patient safety. The goal is to ensure that the knowledge gained through health care research is translated into measurable improvements in the health care system and better care for patients. The products of the Agency include knowledge that supports decisionmaking to improve health care, as well as research-based tools that can help improve quality and reduce costs. For more information on AHRQ's organizational structure and how the Agency functions, see the appendix at the back of this report.

AHRQ's Customers

AHRQ's customers are decisionmakers who need objective, evidence-based, and timely information to make informed decisions about the health care they provide, receive, and purchase. These customers include clinical decisionmakers, health care system decisionmakers, policymakers, and patients.

- **Clinical Decisionmakers.** The evidence uncovered through AHRQ-sponsored research and tools developed from those findings help clinicians, consumers, patients, and health care institutions make informed choices about which treatments work, for whom, when, and at what cost.

- **Health Care System Decisionmakers.** Health plan and health care system managers use the findings and tools developed through AHRQ-sponsored research to make choices on how to improve the health care system's ability to increase access to care and deliver high-quality, high-value care. Purchasers use the products of AHRQ-sponsored research to obtain high-quality health care services.

- **Policymakers.** Public- and private-sector policymakers use the information produced by AHRQ to expand their ability to monitor and evaluate the impact of system changes on outcomes, quality, access, cost, and use of health care and to devise policies designed to improve the performance of the system.

How AHRQ's Research Helps People

Across the Nation, policymakers, clinicians, patients, and consumers are making better-informed, cost-effective health care decisions, and they are receiving higher quality care thanks to AHRQ-supported research. The following are just a few examples of the research AHRQ has sponsored and how the results of that research have been put into practice by policymakers, those who make purchasing decisions, clinicians, patients, and consumers.

Policymakers Use AHRQ Research in Many Ways

In FY 2001, AHRQ responded to more than 2,500 requests for information from Federal, State, and local government officials searching for evidence to inform their decisions. As a scientific research agency, AHRQ's role in responding to these requests is a simple one: to ensure that policymakers have the benefit of our existing knowledge and past experience so that they can make informed decisions.

AHRQ uses a number of approaches in responding to these requests, including:

• Rigorous analyses of the scientific and medical literature.

• Short-term research on the impact of past policy interventions at the Federal and State levels.

• Simulations of the potential impacts of new policy options.

• Other forms of technical assistance.

The following examples represent selected instances in which AHRQ's research has been used by policymakers to improve the functioning of the entire U.S. health care system.

The Centers for Medicare & Medicaid Services (CMS). CMS revised its *Medicare Coverage Issues Manual* to include a national coverage policy permitting coverage for the treatment of actinic keratosis (AK), a common skin lesion. This coverage decision was informed by an AHRQ technology assessment on the natural history and management of actinic keratoses. This assessment suggests that the presence of AKs is associated with the development of squamous cell carcinoma (SCC), and that some SCCs arising from AKs may metastasize. SCC accounts for a large percentage of all non-melanoma skin cancer deaths in the Medicare population. Before the national coverage policy was issued, coverage decisions for AK removal were left up to local Medicare carriers. As a result, many carriers developed AK policies with varying degrees of restriction. The new national policy set by CMS supersedes any policies formerly used by local carriers.

In the last 2 years, AHRQ has prepared nine technology assessments for the Coverage and Analysis Group at CMS. Coverage decisions have been issued on three of these topics. Decisions related to the other six assessments are still pending in CMS. Three additional technology assessments are currently in preparation at AHRQ.

Vitamin D supplements. As a result of an AHRQ-funded study, the State of North Carolina is providing free vitamin D supplementation to breast-fed infants across the State. Researchers at the Center for Education and Research on

Therapeutics (CERTs) at the University of North Carolina (UNC) at Chapel Hill, and Wake Forest University School of Medicine, Winston-Salem, found that many exclusively breast-fed, dark-skinned infants would benefit from vitamin D supplementation. All of the rickets cases among pediatric patients were among black children who were breast-fed and who had not had vitamin D supplements.

The findings from this study resulted in an immediate change in North Carolina's public health practice. The North Carolina Pediatric Society requested that the State distribute a multivitamin supplement free-of-charge to any exclusively breast-fed infant or child 6 weeks of age or older. Funding for the supplements was provided through a Maternal and Child Health Block Grant and distributed through the Supplemental Nutrition Program for Women, Infants and Children. Over a 16-month period, more than 1,500 children received vitamin D supplements at a cost of about $1.50 per month, per child. Fact sheets were developed to help educate parents and clinicians about the need for vitamin D supplementation for breast-fed infants and children.

Using AHRQ's Quality Indicators (QIs) to assess quality of care. The Healthcare Association of New York State (HANYS) uses the QIs from AHRQ's Healthcare Cost and Utilization Project (HCUP) to assess the quality of care delivered by over 200 hospitals in New York State. A number of programs have been implemented to improve healthcare quality based on these assessments. For example, a program was developed to expand awareness of the availability and effectiveness of immunization programs after QI reports showed low rates of adult immunization for pneumonia and influenza. Similarly, when QI reports showed that certain areas of the State had high rates of hospitalization for diabetes-related illnesses, a diabetes center of excellence was established to improve quality of care for patients with diabetes.

AHRQ's Research Findings Help Clinicians and Patients

The pace of medical discovery and innovation has never been greater. But experience has repeatedly demonstrated that great opportunities for improving health, developed through biomedical research, are easily lost if physicians and patients are unable to make the best use of the knowledge in everyday care. These wasted opportunities result in the underuse of effective interventions, continued reliance on outmoded approaches to patient care, and inappropriate use of new and often more expensive interventions.

Failure to understand which services work best, under what circumstances, and for which types of patients contributes to the ever-increasing cost of care, low quality and ineffective care, threats to patient safety, and avoidable loss of lives.

AHRQ's objective is to close that gap by focusing on the effectiveness and cost-effectiveness of health care services and the organization, management, and financing of the health care systems through which these services are delivered. AHRQ's research ultimately assures that patients and society reap the full rewards of basic research and biomedical innovation.

The following examples illustrate how AHRQ-sponsored research has helped patients with chronic diseases become active participants in their care and spend less time in the hospital.

Chronic disease self-management. A disease management program, developed with AHRQ support, has been widely adopted across the United States, as well as in China, England, New Zealand, Australia, Norway, and Sweden. The 5-year research project funded by AHRQ and the State of California demonstrated the benefits of chronic disease self-management in reducing hospitalization among people with multiple chronic conditions. The researchers developed and evaluated a community-based self-management program for chronic illness. More than 1,000 people with heart disease, lung disease, stroke, or arthritis participated in the 6-month trial and were followed for up to 3 years. Patients who completed this study showed significant improvement in exercise, cognitive symptom management, communication with their doctors, self-reported general health, health distress, fatigue, disability, and social/role activity limitations. They also spent fewer days in the hospital. The Department of Veterans Affairs is using the findings from this research, and the course content has been published as a book and made into an audio relaxation tape.

Advance directives to guide end-of-life care. "Let Me Decide" is a comprehensive advance directive that allows individuals and their families to specify a range of health care choices for life-threatening illnesses, cardiac arrest, and nutrition. The tool was developed by researchers at McMaster University through a grant from AHRQ and was based on AHRQ-funded research suggesting that systematic use of such a program could reduce use of health care services without affecting satisfaction or mortality. With more specific information than is sometimes found in generic advance directives, the "Let Me Decide" advance directive contains a personal statement, a definition of terms used in the document, and a health care chart that allows specific decisions regarding levels of care preferences (palliative, limited, surgical, and intensive), as well as the patient's wishes concerning nutrition and cardiac arrest. In addition to the advanced directive, a complete educational package has been created by New Grange Press that consists of a booklet, three videos, a set of slides, research papers, a cassette audio tape, and "Let Me Decide" advance directive forms with instructions. The booklet is available in eight languages, and the video is available in French and English.

AHRQ's Research Findings Help Providers, Consumers, and Purchasers of Care

AHRQ, in conjunction with both public- and private-sector partners, supports a variety of projects that help people make important choices about the health care they receive. For example:

Using the Web to compare nursing homes. The Center for Medicare & Medicaid Services' very popular Web site, NursingHomeCompare—www.medicare.gov/nhcompare/home.asp—grew out of an AHRQ-funded project to develop a consumer information system to help people find data on nursing homes. The site provides detailed information about the performance of every Medicare and Medicaid certified nursing home in the country. Visitors—including patients, families, and clinicians—can compare nursing homes in a specific geographic area by looking at nursing home characteristics (e.g., number of beds, type of ownership), resident characteristics (e.g., percent of residents with pressure sores or urinary incontinence), State inspection results, and nursing staff information (e.g., number of nurses and types of licenses they hold). The site was launched 2 years ago and has an average of 400,000 page views per month.

Tool to help purchasers of health plans. The National Business Coalition for Health (NBCH) has adopted findings from several AHRQ products, including the July 2001 report on *Making Health Care Safer: A Critical Analysis of Patient Safety Practices*, and incorporated them into their 2002 NBCH request for information (RFI), a standard tool that affiliated employers use to solicit potential health plans with which to contract.

9

AHRQ's Research Portfolio

The needs of AHRQ's customers drive the Agency's research agenda and provide the key to our success. We seek input from our customers in a variety of ways, including: the National Advisory Council, meetings with stakeholder groups, *Federal Register* notices, and through comments submitted by the public via the Agency's Web site (www.ahrq.gov).

AHRQ's research agenda is reflected in a variety of activities that together build the infrastructure, tools, and knowledge for measurable improvements in America's health care system. Researchers—including grantees, contractors, and intramural investigators—build on the foundation laid by biomedical science in determining which interventions can work under ideal circumstances. But knowing that these interventions work is only a first step. We also need to make sure that the interventions are used correctly to improve patients' health and that they are effective in everyday practice.

Opportunities for Research

The mission of AHRQ could not be achieved without talented health services researchers who are dedicated to excellence in their own work and the work of their colleagues. They understand the importance of evidence to inform decisionmaking and improve health care quality. In addition to the researchers on AHRQ's staff, about three-quarters of the Agency's budget is awarded as grants and contracts to support the work of researchers at universities, in clinical sites such as hospitals and doctor's offices, and in research institutions.

AHRQ's research funds are awarded either through targeted announcements that address specific research questions or in response to ideas generated by researchers on significant issues in the health care system. Both of these mechanisms—targeted research requests and unsolicited investigator-initiated research proposals—are important and complementary. The Agency's targeted research initiatives respond to the specific needs of individual customers or the needs of the health care system as a whole, although researchers have latitude to design their own projects within the scope of a targeted request.

Unsolicited Research

The topics addressed by unsolicited investigator-initiated research proposals reflect timely issues and ideas from the top health services researchers. Forty-one percent of the grants and cooperative agreements funded by AHRQ in FY 2001 were initiated by individual investigators who developed research proposals within an area of interest to the Agency.

Usually, researchers develop their investigator-initiated proposals in response to program announcements (PAs) that broadly describe the Agency's areas of interest. A PA is a formal statement that invites applications on new or ongoing research topics, usually with multiple application receipt dates. AHRQ issued two new program announcements in FY 2001.

FY 2001 Program Announcements

1. **Impact of Payment and Organization on Cost, Quality, and Equity.** Projects funded under this PA are examining the effects of payment and organizational structures and processes on the cost, quality, and equity of health care.

2. **Patient-Centered Care: Customizing Care to Meet Patients' Needs.** Projects funded under this PA focus on design and evaluation of care processes to empower patients, improve patient-provider interaction, help patients and clinicians navigate through complicated health care systems, and improve access, quality, and outcomes.

Recent Investigator-Initiated Projects

In FY 2001, research funded through unsolicited investigator-initiated grants included many studies to help us understand and reduce costs, improve access to care, and identify ways to achieve better health outcomes.

- **Economic Analysis of Pulmonary Artery Catheter Use, University of Pittsburgh.** The researchers are assessing patient costs and outcomes for two alternative approaches to diagnosing and managing acute respiratory distress syndrome and acute lung injury: the pulmonary artery catheter (PAC) and the central venous catheter (CVC).

- **Maine Lumbar Spine Study, Maine Medical Assessment Foundation.** These researchers are assessing the long-term outcomes of surgical and nonsurgical treatment of two common lumbar spine conditions: herniated intervertebral disc and degenerative spinal stenosis. They will continue the followup of nearly 500 currently enrolled patients to 10 years from initial enrollment, with emphasis on costs to managed care and work-related outcomes, including disability compensation and work status.

- **U.S. Valuation of the EuroQol Group's EQ-5D, University of Arizona.**
Cost-effectiveness analysis (CEA) helps decisionmakers weigh the value of
alternative health care investments. Despite the value of this approach when
health care expenditures are rapidly increasing, the usefulness and comparability
of CEAs are limited by the lack of nationally representative information about
individuals' preferences for health outcomes. This study will obtain such
preferences from a nationally representative sample of the U.S. population. The
study population reflects the increasing demographic diversity of the U.S.
population in the 21st century. The results of this project will help
decisionmakers assess the costs and return on investment of promising new
interventions.

Targeted Research Requests

In FY 2001, quality of care—and in particular patient safety—was the
dominant priority for new research. AHRQ issued a series of solicitations in this
area. These solicitations formed an integrated set of activities to design and test
best practices for reducing errors in various settings of care, develop the science
base to inform these efforts, improve provider education to reduce errors,
capitalize on advances in information technology to translate proven effective
strategies into widespread practice, and build the capacity to further reduce errors.

- **Supporting demonstration projects to report medical errors data.** These
activities include 24 projects for $24.7 million to study different methods of
collecting data on errors or analyzing existing data to identify factors that put
patients at risk of medical errors.

- **Using computers and information technology to prevent medical errors.**
These activities include 22 projects for $5.3 million. The researchers will
develop and test the use of computers and information technology to reduce
medical errors, improve patient safety, and improve quality of care.

- **Understanding the impact of working conditions on patient safety.** These
activities include eight projects for $3 million to examine how staffing, fatigue,
stress, sleep deprivation, and other factors can lead to errors. These issues—
which have been studied extensively in aviation, manufacturing, and other
industries—have not be closely examined in health care settings. [Note: In all,
AHRQ allocated about $10 million in FY 2001 to working conditions and
health care quality.]

- **Developing innovative approaches to improving patient safety.** These
activities include 23 projects for $8 million to research and develop innovative
approaches to improving patient safety at health care facilities and organizations
in geographically diverse locations across the country.

- **Disseminating research results.** These activities include seven projects for $2.4 million to help educate clinicians and others about the results of patient safety research. This work will help develop, demonstrate, and evaluate new approaches to improving provider education in order to reduce errors, such as applying new knowledge on patient safety to curricula development, continuing education, simulation models, and other provider training strategies.

- **Other patient safety research initiatives.** These include 10 other projects for $6.4 million that will expand the evidence base on what works and doesn't work in improving safety; support meetings of State and local officials to advance local patient safety initiatives; help small businesses explore new products to help improve safety; assess the feasibility of implementing a patient safety improvement corps; and carry out other patient safety initiatives.

Examples of Targeted Research

- **Consumer Assessment of Health Plans II (CAHPS®II).** This request for applications (RFA), issued in late FY 2001, provides support for projects to expand CAHPS and enhance the usefulness of CAHPS products. Awards under this project are expected in spring 2002.

- **Research Infrastructure and Capacity.** Nine projects were funded for nearly $3 million to build and strengthen the Nation's research infrastructure, particularly those entities that serve racial/ethnic minorities, and broaden the geographic distribution of health services research funding. The projects were funded under two AHRQ research infrastructure development initiatives announced in FY 2001: the Minority Research Infrastructure Support Program (M-RISP), and the Building Research Infrastructure and Capacity (BRIC) Program. See page 44 for examples of BRIC projects.

Building the Research Infrastructure

AHRQ contributes to excellence in health care delivery through research conducted by a cadre of well-trained and talented health services researchers. To maintain and nurture this vital resource, the Agency supports a variety of training and career development opportunities through individual and institutional grant programs. In FY 2001, AHRQ provided support for 232 trainees through these programs:

- Dissertation research support.

- Predoctoral fellowships for minority students.

- National Research Service Awards (pre- and postdoctoral fellowships), including both institutional and individual programs.

- Independent Scientist Awards (K awards).

Investing in development of the research infrastructure—including training of new investigators—is fundamental to producing the next generation of health services researchers. These investments also return a more immediate payoff in the form of high-quality research. The products and lessons learned from such research are useful to regional, State, and national decisionmakers in assessing the effectiveness of current programs and planning for future policies that address the costs and financing of health care, the use of health care services, and access to care across diverse regions and populations.

Investments in Training

An integral component of AHRQ's training efforts is support for fellowships and dissertation research. Many trainees are focusing on issues related to managed care, Medicare and Medicaid, and health care costs, including the costs of prescription medicines. Examples of AHRQ-supported dissertation research and fellowships include:

- **Quality-adjusted cost functions for HMOs.** This researcher is examining how the quality of services provided by HMOs affects the cost to enrollees and whether there are financial paybacks to organizations that invest in quality.

- **Impact of managed care on minority physicians and patients.** This trainee is investigating the effects of managed care contracting on access to minority providers and the use of health services by minority patients, who tend to rely heavily on minority providers.

- **Effects of public insurance on dental health outcomes.** This researcher is comparing children's dental health status and receipt of services through two State-sponsored programs in North Carolina: Health Choice, which provides dental services through the State's private Blue Cross/Blue Shield program, and the State Medicaid program. The goal is to determine the benefits of public dental insurance for low-income children when it is structured similar to private insurance.

- **Medical group response to HMO selective contracting.** This trainee is focusing on managed care selective contracting and how it is affected by market power and State policies such as those broadening the rights of patients to choose their health care providers.

- **Effects of drug advertising on prescription choice.** The goal of this study is to examine the effects of direct-to-consumer drug advertising on prescription drug choices and costs. The student hopes to determine the extent to which such advertising undermines insurers' efforts to induce price sensitivity in prescribing behavior.

- **Effects of WIC on children's Medicaid dental use and costs.** This researcher is looking at the relationship between the Women, Infants, and Children Supplemental Food Program (WIC) on use of oral health care services and costs to the Medicaid program for children under 5 years of age.

Additional information on all of the Agency's funding opportunities—including an ongoing program announcement that describes the priorities for investigator-initiated research, targeted initiatives, and career-related grant programs—is available at www.ahrq.gov/fund.

15

Partnerships and Coordination

Collaboration allows organizations to make progress and achieve results far beyond what they could do as individual groups. Two or more organizations can leverage their resources by working together on projects of mutual interest. AHRQ works in partnership with many other agencies and organizations to pool ideas and resources in research and dissemination. Our partner organizations include the various HHS agencies, other components of the Federal government, State and local governments, and private-sector organizations, all of whom help us achieve our goals.

Most of these partnerships are related to the development of new knowledge, development of tools and other decision-support mechanisms, and/or the translation of research findings into practice. Examples of this collaboration include efforts to:

1. Develop new knowledge through research.

   - AHRQ co-funds individual research projects and sponsors joint research solicitations with other HHS agencies.

   - In FY 2001, AHRQ and the Kaiser Family Foundation completed a random national survey of more than 2,000 adults to determine how consumers judge health care quality. The survey, "Americans as Health Care consumers: The role of Quality Information," was developed and sponsored jointly by AHRQ and the Kaiser Family Foundation.

2. Develop tools, measures, and decision-support mechanisms.

   - Many agencies (e.g., the National Institutes of Health, the Centers for Medicare & Medicaid Services, and the Department of Veterans Affairs) are working closely with AHRQ's evidence-based practice centers (EPCs) to develop assessments of existing scientific evidence to guide their work.

   - Evidence reports prepared by AHRQ-supported EPCs are being used in the development of clinical practice guidelines by a number of private-sector organizations, including the American Psychiatric Association, the American Academy of Pediatrics, the American Heart Association, and many others.

16

3. Translate research into practice.

- A number of companies and organizations have joined AHRQ in disseminating smoking cessation materials. These include the American Cancer Society, the American Academy of Pediatrics, and the Michigan Department of Community Health.

4. Coordinate patient safety activities.

- In FY 2001, AHRQ joined other Department of Health and Human Services agencies as a member of the new HHS Patient Safety Task Force. The Federal agencies leading this effort include AHRQ, the Centers for Disease Control and Prevention (CDC), the Food and Drug Administration (FDA), and the Centers for Medicare & Medicaid Services (CMS). The goal is to work closely with the States and private sector in this effort and to improve existing systems to collect data on patient safety. The Patient Safety Task Force will study how to implement a user-friendly, Internet-based patient safety reporting format to enable faster cross-matching and electronic analysis of data and more rapid responses to patient safety problems.

Working in partnership:

- HRSA and AARP partnered with AHRQ to develop the Put Prevention into Practice personal health guide for adults over 50.

- The Healthcare Cost and Utilization Project (HCUP) is a long-standing public-private partnership between AHRQ and 25 partner States to build a multistate data system.

- Thanks to partnerships between AHRQ and 14 companies/organizations (e.g., Midwest Business Group on Health, IBM, United Parcel Service, and others), we have been able to greatly enhance dissemination of our Quality Navigational Tool, a guidebook to help individuals apply research findings on quality measures and make major decisions about health plans, doctors, treatments, hospitals, and long-term care.

Strategic Goals and Performance Planning

Strategic Planning at AHRQ

The AHRQ strategic plan guides the overall management of the Agency, and it serves as a road map for AHRQ activities during the year. Each year, during planning and budget development activities, we assess the progress the Agency has made toward achieving each of the goals and plan for work in years to come. The program performance information that follows here is arrayed according to our strategic plan goals and is consistent with the requirements of the Government Performance and Results Act of 1993 (GPRA).

Goal 1: Support Improvements in Health Outcomes. This goal focuses on research to understand and improve decisionmaking at all levels of the health care system, the outcomes of health care, and in particular, what works, for whom, when, and at what cost.

Selected highlights from AHRQ funded evidence reports or technology assessments that are relevant for State or Federal health policy decisions follow.

- Evidence from a review of the impact of behavioral interventions on dietary outcomes considered to be relevant to cancer risk—such as dietary fat intake and consumption of fruits and vegetables—was incorporated into a review for the National Cancer Policy Board (a joint National Cancer Institute (NCI/Institute of Medicine (IOM) collaboration). In addition, the NCI has broadly disseminated the evidence report, posted a link to the report on its Web site, and highlighted the evidence at a variety of investigator meetings, including the American Institute for Cancer Research conference.

- A recent review of studies that compared conventional and newer Pap tests with the current standard found that, although the conventional Pap test is only moderately accurate, serial testing (Pap testing every 3 to 5 years) will probably detect abnormalities missed in one screening because cervical cancer usually is a slow-growing disease, and many low-grade lesions regress spontaneously. Findings from this report have been considered by two large HMOs—Excellus Healthcare (Blue Cross/Blue Shield of upstate New York) and Henry Ford (Detroit)—to develop coverage policies with respect to cervical cancer screening using new liquid-based technologies. In addition, the cost-effectiveness model from this report is being used by a major pharmaceutical company to assist in the planning and evaluation of a human papillomavirus virus (HPV) vaccine, and the U.S. Preventive Services Task Forces used the evidence in the formulation of its recommendations on cervical cancer screening.

- Research showed that routine medical testing prior to cataract surgery does not improve outcomes and in most cases is unnecessary.

Goal 2: Strengthen Quality Measurement and Improvement. This goal involves support for research to develop valid and reproducible measures of the processes and outcomes of care, studies to identify the causes of medical errors and ways to prevent them, research to develop strategies for incorporating quality improvement measures into programs, and studies on dissemination and implementation of validated quality improvement measures and tools.

These examples illustrate how findings from AHRQ research have been used by our public and private partners.

- The American Academy of Pediatrics developed a clinical practice guideline on treatment of attention deficit and hyperactivity disorder based on our evidence report on the same topic.

- The Centers for Medicare & Medicaid Services used U.S. Preventive Services Task Force recommendations to develop messages for consumers and clinicians regarding Medicare-covered services for osteoporosis, cervical cancer, prostate cancer, and breast cancer.

- The American Society of Adolescent Medicine used the AHRQ evidence report on pharmacotherapy for alcohol dependence as the basis for their guideline on the same topic.

- Research sponsored by AHRQ found that the antifungal medication fluconazole may help prevent the development of thrush (a disorder caused by infection of the mouth with yeast) in the mouths of HIV-infected patients.

Goal 3: Identify Strategies to Improve Access, Foster Appropriate Use, and Reduce Unnecessary Expenditures. In working toward this goal, we support research to identify ways to enhance access to care, particularly for vulnerable populations; determine what works and doesn't work in health care to ensure the appropriate use of services; and develop new ways to promote cost-effectiveness in the use of scarce health care resources.

Examples of AHRQ research findings at work include:

- The Healthcare Association of New York and the Texas Health Care Information Council disseminated data from AHRQ's Healthcare Cost and Utilization Project (HCUP) that led regional hospitals to reform internal practices, form collaborations to improve quality of care, and inform the public about variations in certain treatment patterns or medical procedures, such as heart bypass surgery and cesarean deliveries.

- AHRQ's research portfolio on low-income populations has informed the work of the Health Resources and Services Administration (HRSA) on evaluating and improving the health care safety net. In addition, our research has played an important role in the Centers for Disease Control's Free Vaccine Program, which supports the delivery of immunizations in primary care settings.

Goal 1 – Outcomes

Outcomes Research Portfolio

For more than a decade, AHRQ has been supporting research on the outcomes and effectiveness of health care. Outcomes research provides evidence about the benefits, risks, and results of treatments so clinicians and patients can make more informed health care choices. Outcomes research answers a number of very basic questions about the health care system: What works and doesn't work? Is it having the desired effect? Does it provide value for the money spent? The answers to these questions form a solid foundation for efforts to improve health care quality and patient safety, enhance access to care, and improve the cost-effectiveness of care.

In addition, outcomes research also examines variations in care from one part of the country to another and from one population group to another. Time and again, studies have documented that therapies as commonplace as hysterectomy and hernia repair are performed much more frequently in some regions than in others, even when there is no difference in the underlying rates of disease. By linking the care people get to the outcomes they experience, outcomes research has become the key to developing better ways to monitor and improve the quality of care provided in hospitals, physicians' offices, and other health care settings.

The results of AHRQ-funded outcomes research (e.g., quality measures and other tools) are becoming part of the "report cards" that purchasers and consumers can use to assess the quality of care provided in health plans. For public programs such as Medicaid and Medicare, outcomes research provides policymakers with the tools to monitor and improve quality, both in traditional health plans and in managed care.

In FY 2001, AHRQ's outcomes research portfolio included more than 70 ongoing projects that focused on a wide range of topics, as well as a number of flagship programs such as the Centers for Education and Research on Therapeutics (CERTs), Evidence-based Practice Centers (EPCs), and the U.S. Preventive Services Task Force (USPSTF).

Examples of findings from recent AHRQ-supported outcomes research include:

- **Otitis media.** Each year, about 280,000 children under age 3 with persistent fluid and inflammation of the middle ear have tubes inserted in their ears—a procedure called tympanostomy. Now, an AHRQ-supported study has found that in most cases, tympanostomy does not measurably improve children's

21

speech, language, cognitive abilities, or psychosocial development up to age 3. The study enrolled 588 infants and followed them to age 3.

- **Community-acquired pneumonia.** More than 2 million cases of community-acquired pneumonia (CAP) are diagnosed each year in the United States, resulting in about 10 million physician visits, 500,000 hospitalizations, and 45,000 deaths, making it one of the leading causes of mortality and health care expenditures for Medicare beneficiaries. AHRQ-supported researchers developed a Pneumonia Severity Index (PSI) to identify which patients were most at risk of dying from CAP and demonstrated its validity to guide decisions made by clinicians, patients, and families about which patients need hospitalization and which patients can be safely treated at home. In related work, the investigators found that adding one blood test further enhances this decision. For patients who are hospitalized, the investigators evaluated when patients can be safely switched to oral antibiotics to decrease the length of stay. The investigators are now working with quality improvement organizations in Pennsylvania and Connecticut to improve clinical decisions about hospitalization and improve quality of care for Medicare beneficiaries.

- **Lower respiratory tract infection in nursing home residents.** Lower respiratory tract infection is a leading cause of hospitalization and mortality in nursing home residents. Moreover, it is difficult to accurately diagnose in individuals who have multiple chronic illnesses and atypical findings. An AHRQ-supported study evaluated over 1,400 episodes of lower respiratory infections in 36 Missouri nursing homes and developed a tool that can help clinicians determine which patients have severe infections and need to be hospitalized and which can be safely treated in the nursing home, thus avoiding discomfort and complications.

- **Cost-effective approaches to improve detection and management of depression.** Depression is a leading cause of decreased function and time lost from work. Multiple studies have found that the majority of clinically depressed patients are not identified; for those who are detected, treatment often is inadequate. An AHRQ-supported study to improve quality of care for depressed patients substantially increased both detection and adequate treatment rates. The intervention was designed to fit the circumstances and coverage of individual practices and patients (rather than a 'one size fits all' approach). At the end of 2 years, patients receiving care in diverse health care settings who participated in the quality improvement program were more likely to have their symptoms recognized, received more appropriate treatment, returned to normal function more rapidly, and missed less time from work than those who received usual care. This intervention was found to be both cost effective and straightforward to implement in other settings. The research team developed tools for broad use in health care organizations, and they have received thousands of inquiries for these materials.

U.S. Preventive Services Task Force

The U.S. Preventive Services Task Force (USPSTF) is another critical source of information on what does and does not work in the health care system specific to clinical prevention. First convened in 1984, the USPSTF is an independent panel of health care experts. The Task Force is charged with evaluating the scientific evidence for the effectiveness of a range of clinical preventive services—including common screening tests, counseling for health behavior change, and chemoprevention—and producing age- and risk-factor-specific recommendations for these services. The Task Force published its first set of recommendations in the 1989 *Guide to Clinical Preventive Services*, which was revised in 1995.

The third USPSTF was convened in early FY 1999 and began work on 12 initial topics selected by Task Force members based on preliminary work by two of AHRQ's Evidence-based Practice Centers: the Research Triangle Institute/University of North Carolina at Chapel Hill and the Oregon Health & Science University. The selection process included a preliminary literature search of new information on prevention and screening published since 1995; consultation with professional societies, health care organizations, and outside prevention experts; a review of current levels of controversy and variations in practice; and consideration of the potential for a change from the 1995 USPSTF recommendations.

The 12 topics are:

- Chemoprevention (for example, tamoxifen and related drugs) to prevent breast cancer (new topic).

- Vitamin supplementation to prevent cancer or coronary heart disease (vitamin E, folate, beta carotene, and vitamin C) (new topic).

- Screening for bacterial vaginosis in pregnancy (new topic).

- Developmental screening in children (new topic).

- Screening for diabetes mellitus (updated topic).

- Newborn hearing screening (updated topic).

- Screening for skin cancer (updated topic).

- Counseling to prevent unintended pregnancy (updated topic).

- Screening for high cholesterol (updated topic).

- Postmenopausal hormone therapy (updated topic).

- Screening for chlamydial infection (updated topic).

- Screening for depression (updated topic).

In FY 2001, the third USPSTF issued its first four recommendations covering chlamydia screening, lipid screening, skin cancer, and bacterial vaginosis.

Chlamydia screening. The Task Force recommended that primary care clinicians screen all sexually active women ages 25 and younger for chlamydia, as well as older women who are at risk for chlamydia, as part of regular health care visits.

Chlamydia is the most common bacterial sexually transmitted disease in the United States, with an estimated 3 million new cases each year. Most women have no symptoms when initially infected, but if they go untreated, they can develop pelvic inflammatory disease, infertility, and other serious health problems, including increased risk of HIV infection. Treatment with antibiotics is easy and effective.

Lipid screening. In a broadening of its 1996 recommendations, the USPSTF recommended that regular screening for high blood cholesterol and other lipid abnormalities, which can lead to coronary heart disease, should not have an upper age limit (previously set by the panel at age 65).

The USPSTF also issued a new recommendation calling for the screening of younger adults for lipid abnormalities beginning at age 20 if they have risk factors for coronary heart disease such as diabetes, family history of heart disease, tobacco use, or high blood pressure. In addition, the panel revised its 1996 statement to recommend that for initial screening purposes, clinicians measure high density lipoprotein (HDL) cholesterol along with total cholesterol.

Skin cancer. The Task Force concluded, based on its most recent review of the literature, that there is still insufficient scientific evidence to determine whether regular total body skin examination for skin cancer is effective in reducing illness and death. This is the same conclusion the Task Force reached in 1996.

Bacterial vaginosis. Bacterial vaginosis is a common condition among women of childbearing age that results in a vaginal discharge caused by an imbalance in vaginal bacteria. Despite research showing that pregnant women with bacterial vaginosis have a higher risk of preterm delivery, the Task Force has concluded that the evidence does not merit regular screening for bacterial vaginosis in all pregnant women as an effective way to reduce the incidence of preterm delivery.

For women at high risk due to a previous preterm delivery, however, the USPSTF found conflicting results regarding the benefit of screening and treatment and concluded that these options be left to the discretion of clinicians.

The USPSTF conducts impartial assessments of scientific evidence for a broad range of clinical conditions to produce recommendations for the regular provision of clinical preventive services. The Task Force grades the strength of evidence, as follows: A (strongly recommends), B (recommends), C (makes no recommendation for or against), D (recommends against), and I (insufficient evidence to recommend for or against). As the panel updates the 70 chapters in its 1996 report, it is issuing revised recommendations as they are completed on the AHRQ Web site, the National Guideline Clearinghouse, and in medical journals. Releasing the recommendations as they are finished rather than all at once, as in the past, will get them into the hands of clinicians more quickly.

Put Prevention Into Practice

AHRQ's Put Prevention Into Practice (PPIP) program helps translate the evidence-based recommendations of the U.S. Preventive Services Task Force into practice through the development and dissemination of resources for providers, patients, and office systems. PPIP emphasizes the importance of a comprehensive, system-wide, team approach to delivering effective preventive interventions. AHRQ works closely with public and private partners to disseminate PPIP resources. PPIP materials include information on preventive services recommendations; an implementation guide, including flowsheets and other forms; and personal health guides for children, adults, and people over 50.

During FY 2001—in conjunction with the release by the third USPSTF of its recommendations on screening for chlamydia, lipid disorders, bacterial vaginosis in pregnancy, and skin cancer—work was completed on a new information kit, *What's New in Clinical Prevention?* The kit includes factsheets on the newly released topics and other information to promote the Task Force and PPIP. In addition, a prevention LISTSERV® was established.

During FY 2001, work was completed on *A Step-by-Step Guide to Delivering Clinical Preventive Services: A Systems Approach.* The guide describes easy to follow, logical steps to develop a formal system for delivering clinical preventive services. It is based on scientific and empirical evidence and has been found effective in many settings. The new guide breaks the process into small, manageable tasks;

25

> ## Texas uses PPIP in clinical practice
>
> The Texas Department of Health has implemented PPIP in various clinical settings throughout the State. They organized a PPIP central office to provide oversight and trained regional public health nurses to provide technical assistance. The nurses work with individual sites to assess readiness, ensure that PPIP tools are used effectively, monitor chart documentation, and help the sites link with local resources for referrals. The central office focuses on promoting quality assurance, developing prevention systems and materials, and providing guidance to clinicians, not only in Texas but in other parts of the country as well.
>
> Examples of specialized PPIP tools developed by Texas include:
>
> - Health risk profile that identifies genetic, behavioral, and environmental risk factors.
>
> - Readiness tool that can be used to assess readiness of a clinical practice to implement PPIP.
>
> - Patient education materials on primary prevention for various health risks.
>
> - Policies and procedures manual that helps individual practices design tailored PPIP systems.

provides tools for tracking the delivery of preventive care, such as flowsheets and health risk profiles; includes worksheets and templates; and identifies resources for more information.

Centers for Education and Research on Therapeutics

Neither patients nor their caregivers should have to guess which therapies are the best or live in fear that a mistake will be made in treatment. This is the basis of AHRQ's Centers for Education and Research on Therapeutics (CERTs) program. AHRQ was given authority to support the CERTs initiative under the Food and Drug Modernization Act of 1997. Between 1999 and 2000, AHRQ established seven centers under the CERTs program, each of which focuses on therapies used in a particular population or therapeutic area. The CERTs conduct research and provide education that will advance the optimal use of drugs, medical devices, and biological products.

The U.S. system of developing and marketing medical products, which requires that adequate and well-controlled studies show that products are safe and effective for their intended use, has produced great benefits. The system does have some drawbacks, however. Although drugs, medical devices, and biological products

Focus of Centers for Education and Research on Therapeutics (CERTs)

- Duke University: Approved drugs and therapeutic devices in cardiovascular medicine.

- Georgetown University: Reduction of drug interactions, particularly in women.

- University of North Carolina: Rational use of therapeutics in pediatric populations.

- Vanderbilt University: Prescription medication use in the Medicaid managed care population.

- HMO Research Network: Use of large managed care databases to study prescribing patterns, dosing outcomes, and policy input.

- University of Pennsylvania: Antibiotic drug resistance, drug use, and intervention studies.

- University of Alabama: Therapeutics for musculoskeletal disorders.

improve health for thousands of people, side effects, misuse, and overuse of products seriously impair the health of many others. The fact is that many patients potentially could benefit from a therapy but do not receive it; this may be through lack of information, oversight, or in the mistaken belief that the therapy will do them harm. In addition, studies may not test medical products in combination with other therapies often used by the same patients. Further, once approved, drugs and devices often are used for purposes other than those for which they were approved—sometimes these uses are supported by studies, but not always. Finally, some side effects of medical products emerge only after they have been approved for sale, when large numbers of people begin to use them.

The CERTs program aims to fill these information gaps by answering important questions that have not been addressed; provide results, positive or negative, for all to see; and strive to develop a learning curriculum for current and future caregivers. Finally, the CERTs program represents a major step toward giving people the information they need to make the best choices possible. The participants in the CERTs program—Federal government agencies, academic organizations, managed care organizations, drug and device companies, practitioners, commercial research groups, and consumer groups, among others—have voluntarily committed to seeking answers together, putting society's interests first.

Following are a few examples of how the CERTs serve as a trusted national resource for people seeking to improve health through the best use of medical therapies.

- The University of North Carolina (UNC) CERT developed and implemented an adverse drug event (ADE) reporting system for hospitalized infants, children, and adolescents. Over a 14-month period, pediatric ADE reporting jumped 500 percent to an average of nearly six reports per day. More than 70 percent of the reports involved only potential ADEs, such as prescribing an incorrect dose, that never reached the patient because a nurse or pharmacist intervened. The program has been so successful that it is being expanded to all patient-care areas at UNC.

- The costs of antibiotic resistance are very high, both in financial and human terms. Estimates range from $75 million to $7.5 billion for costs related to resistant infections, which carry at least twice the risk of serious illness and hospitalization as infections that respond to drugs. For example, patients with acne often take oral antibiotics for many years, but the effects of these drugs on the patients and their families are not well understood. The University of Pennsylvania CERT is carrying out case-control and observational cohort studies to examine the possible link between long-term tetracycline use for acne and the development of both antibiotic resistance and infections.

- Some commonly prescribed drugs can affect the electrical properties of the heart and may trigger life-threatening arrhythmias. The Vanderbilt University CERT considered the class of drugs called antipsychotics, which are used to treat schizophrenia and other serious mental illnesses. Compared with people who had never used these medicines, those who were taking high doses were more than twice as likely to die suddenly from cardiac causes. For patients who had severe cardiovascular disease, rates of sudden cardiac death were more than three times higher among those who took antipsychotics. Even among those with moderate or mild heart disease, rates of sudden cardiac death were proportionally higher among patients who took antipsychotics compared with those who didn't.

Evidence-based Practice Centers

AHRQ's 12 Evidence-based Practice Centers (EPCs) develop evidence reports and technology assessments on therapies and technologies that are common, expensive, and/or significant for the Medicare and Medicaid populations. The EPCs systematically review and analyze the published scientific literature to develop the reports. During their reviews, the EPCs flag areas where the evidence base is sparse and suggest future research directions.

> **Examples of FY 2001 AHRQ-Funded EPC Reports and Technology Assessments**
>
> - Effect of seasonal allergies on working populations
> - Management of venous thrombosis
> - Use of glycohemoglobin and microalbuminuria in diagnosis and monitoring of diabetes mellitus
> - Neonatal hyperbilirubinemia
> - Hyperbaric oxygen therapy for brain injury and stroke
> - Vaginal birth following c-section
> - Effect of patient safety on health care working conditions
> - Management of bronchiolitis
> - Management of coronary heart disease in women
> - Making health care safer: Critical analysis of patient safety practices

Since 1997, the EPCs have conducted more than 80 systematic reviews and analyses of the literature on a wide spectrum of topics, and they have incorporated the results and conclusions into evidence reports and technology assessments. Some of these reviews are ongoing, and others have been published.

Potential users of these reports and assessments include doctors, medical and professional associations, health system managers, researchers, consumer organizations, and policymakers. These public- and private-sector organizations use the reports as the basis for developing their own clinical guidelines, performance measures, and other quality improvement tools and strategies. The reports and assessments often are used in formulating reimbursement and coverage policies. All EPCs collaborate with other medical and research organizations so that a broad range of experts can be included in the development process.

Nominations of topics are solicited routinely through notices in the *Federal Register* and are accepted on an ongoing basis. Professional organizations, health plans, providers, and others who nominate topics are considered partners and agree to use the evidence reports when they are completed. AHRQ invites comments from interested parties about the EPC program with respect to what has worked well, what has not worked well, and what changes and improvements could be made. We also are interested in suggestions about new opportunities, such as what steps the Agency can take to encourage more health care organizations and other relevant groups to translate EPC reports into clinical practice guidelines and related products.

AHRQ funded 28 new evidence topics in FY 2001. Seven of the topics were nominated by private-sector professional societies and providers, and two are part of AHRQ's patient safety initiative. Nineteen EPC reports were funded by other

Federal agencies. One EPC found that bone density measured at the hip by dual energy x-ray absorptiometry (DXA) is the best predictor of hip fracture, and that repeating the bone density tests within the first year of treatment is not recommended. This finding is particularly important to the estimated 14 million American women over age 50 who are affected by low bone density at the hip. Another EPC found that a synthetic hormone developed to replace a natural hormone was effective in reducing the need for transfusions in cancer patients with anemia resulting from chemotherapy.

National Guideline Clearinghouse

The National Guideline Clearinghouse™ (NGC) is an Internet resource for evidence-based clinical practice guidelines. It has been operational for 3 years and now contains more than 1,000 clinical practice guidelines. The NGC was developed by AHRQ in partnership with the American Medical Association (AMA) and the American Association of Health Plans (AAHP) to be a resource for physicians, nurses, educators, and other health care professionals.

NGC Helps Disseminate Guidelines

The University of Michigan Health System (UMHS) in Ann Arbor has developed a program known as Guidelines Utilization, Implementation, Development, and Evaluation Studies (GUIDES). Now in its sixth year, UMHS has 10 of its guidelines in the National Guideline Clearinghouse.

In responding to a recent survey of NGC, UMHS called the NGC especially valuable in disseminating their work and a wonderful enhancement to their existing processes.

Guidelines for the NGC site are submitted by over 165 health care organizations and other entities. New guidelines are added weekly. Over the past 3 years, NGC has had more than 4 million visitors, processed over 40 million requests, and received more than 81 million hits. More than 46,000 users visit the NGC each week.

AHRQ does not require users of the National Guideline Clearinghouse to register in order to use the site. However, AHRQ recently completed the second customer satisfaction survey of NGC, which does provide some insight into who uses the site. Physicians represented the largest portion of survey respondents (40.6 percent), followed by nurses and/or nurse practitioners (18.9 percent). More than 93 percent of respondents rated their overall satisfaction with NGC as either "fairly satisfied" or "very satisfied" compared with 89 percent for the first annual survey. Respondents also provided many useful comments on how they were using the site in their clinical work.

Goal 2 – Quality

Making Quality Count

Millions of Americans receive high-quality health care services. The United States has many of the world's finest health care professionals, academic health care centers, and other institutions. Yet, too often, patients receive substandard care. Sometimes they receive too many services or unnecessary services that undermine the quality of care and needlessly increase costs. At other times they do not receive needed services that have been proven to be effective.

The research that provided much of the basis for the 2001 report by the Institute of Medicine (IOM), *Crossing the Quality Chasm*, goes back several decades to early studies on quality of care, most of which were supported by AHRQ and its predecessor agencies. In its report, the IOM pointed out that quality problems occur across all types of cancer care and in all aspects of the process of care. For example, the IOM report described "underuse of mammography for early cancer detection, lack of adherence to standards for diagnosis, inadequate patient counseling regarding treatment options, and underuse of radiation therapy and adjuvant chemotherapy following surgery."

Poor quality care leads to patients who are sicker, have more disabilities, incur higher costs, and have lower confidence in the Nation's health care system. There is great potential to improve the quality of health care provided to Americans, and AHRQ is committed to this goal. We are working to develop and test measures of quality, identify the best ways to collect, compare, and communicate data on quality, and widely disseminate information about effective strategies to improve the quality of care.

Following are examples of AHRQ-supported research now in progress that focuses on improving health care quality:

- Harvard University researchers are assessing the quality of care provided to HIV patients by clinics receiving Title III Ryan White funds, changes in care subsequent to quality training, and the organizational characteristics and policies that facilitate or hinder such changes, such as providers' attitudes and beliefs, formal training, knowledge, and experience. They will assess the effects of an intensive quality improvement project involving multiple HIV care sites and identify clinician and clinic characteristics that predict the most improvement and sustained change.

- Diabetes affects 10 million patients, costs $100 billion annually, and causes significant complications, including vision problems, kidney problems, problems with the nervous system, and cardiovascular disease. In this 3-year project underway at the University of Chicago, researchers are testing two models of quality improvement applied to diabetes care in community health centers (CHCs): one, a collaborative approach including intensive, extended training in total quality management and a chronic disease model; and two, a control model consisting of basic brief training in total quality management and a chronic disease model. The long-term goal is to improve the quality of care and outcomes of poor, vulnerable patients with diabetes who receive their care at rural and urban CHCs, which are critical sites of primary care for 10 million Americans who reside in medically underserved areas.

- A quality improvement study on identifying and treating dangerous levels of jaundice in newborns has contributed to the issuance of a guideline by the American Academy of Pediatrics, which has been advising the research effort. In addition, the Joint Commission on Accreditation of Healthcare Organizations has issued a "sentinel event alert," suggesting that many gaps in quality of care can be seen as patient safety issues. Jaundice is a very frequent condition in newborns that, rarely, can become a devastating illness called kernicterus, producing levels of developmental disability that may not be apparent for months or years. Jaundice occurs when the developing liver produces levels of bilirubin beyond the ability of the infant's body to process, damaging the brain. The condition is also related to dehydration, gastroenteritis, and inadequate nutrition. Shorter hospital stays are thought to create discontinuities in care that occur just when bilirubin levels may be peaking. The researchers are attempting to find feasible and effective interventions that will ensure reliable identification and treatment of dangerous bilirubin levels. The study, which will use this condition to explore quality improvement in complex health care organizations, is being carried out in cooperation with Blue-Cross-Blue Shield of Texas and the Henry Ford Health System.

Examples of recent findings from AHRQ-supported research on improving health care quality include:

- Researchers at the University of Alabama have developed and tested a straightforward statistical method for creating quality benchmarks that respond to both level and volume of performance. The method, called Achievable Benchmarks of Care (ABCs), reduces the influence of apparent high performers, such as physicians, whose ratings apply to very small numbers. If a physician were to have only one diabetic patient, for example, performing a foot exam on that single patient might not be a good indication of routinely high quality. The artificially high indicator, if it became the benchmark, was thought to reduce the motivation of other physicians to attain the benchmark level. ABCs have been tested in feedback to physicians on care for diabetes and several other conditions. In most cases, ABCs have been shown to result in improved quality.

- A catalogue has been developed of over 300 quality indicators for mental health and substance abuse services, providing information on the evidence base and the current users of these methods. The Harvard-based researchers have designed a system for Web access for service providers looking to improve the quality of care they deliver.

- When county emergency medical service (EMS) administrators in Southern California decided to include airway intubation for children among the procedures used by paramedics on ambulances, as it is for adults, they sought out a pediatric emergency physician from the Harbor-UCLA Medical Center in Torrance and asked her to develop a training program for the paramedics. As she examined the task, she became aware that there was no evidence that intubation was an effective replacement for bag-valve-mask resuscitation for children in respiratory distress. Working with all the ambulance providers in Los Angeles and Orange Counties, the researcher developed a plan for a randomized, controlled trial, which was carried out with support from the Health Resources and Services Administration and the Agency for Healthcare Research and Quality. The study found that in comparison with the bag-valve-mask method, intubation did not improve outcomes, had a high risk of error, and seemed of questionable value for children in ambulances. The county has revised its plans, and EMS providers nationally have taken these findings into account in administering their systems.

Using Research Findings to Improve Quality of Care

Thousands of Medicare patients with atrial fibrillation (AF) can benefit from a new quality improvement tool developed with support from AHRQ. Findings from a second study can be used to improve end-of-life care by encouraging more discussions between terminally ill HIV patients and their doctors.

Atrial fibrillation. Researchers found that their new CHADS2 method for predicting risk of stroke in patients with AF is more accurate than existing methods. CHADS2 may be especially helpful for identifying low-risk patients who, by taking aspirin, can avoid the office visits, expense, and risks associated with warfarin, which carries a risk of bleeding.

End-of-life discussions. Half of all HIV-infected people in the United States—especially blacks, Hispanics, injection drug users, and people with low education—never talk about end-of-life care with their doctors. Such discussions could improve physicians' understanding of the types of care their patients want when they are very ill and close to death, and they may lead to designation of a surrogate to make decisions when the patient is too ill to do so.

Patient Safety and Reducing Errors in Medicine

The November 1999 report of the Institute of Medicine (IOM), *To Err is Human: Building a Safer Health System*, focused a great deal of attention on the issues of medical errors and patient safety and showed that a wide gap exists in the quality of care people receive and the quality of care that we as a Nation are capable of providing. The report indicated that as many as 44,000 to 98,000 people die in hospitals each year as at the result of medical errors. Even using the lower estimate, this would make medical errors the eighth leading cause of death in this country.

More people die from medical errors than from automobile accidents (43,458), breast cancer (42,297), or AIDS (16,516). It is estimated that about 7,000 people each year die from medication errors alone—about 16 percent more deaths than the number attributable to work-related injuries.

Although the increased public attention on this issue is a recent phenomenon, AHRQ has recognized for some time that reducing medical errors is critically

Americans are very concerned about medical errors. According to a national poll conducted by the National Patient Safety Foundation:

- 42 percent of respondents had been affected by a medical error, either personally or through a friend or relative.

- 32 percent of the respondents indicated that the error had a permanent negative effect on the patient's health.

The results of an AHRQ/Kaiser Family Foundation survey found that more than 60 percent of the respondents believe there is a role for government in promoting, monitoring, and providing information about the quality of care provided by doctors, hospitals, and health plans.

important for improving the quality of health care. In 1993, the Agency published one of the first reports focused on medical errors. This landmark report noted that 78 percent of adverse drug reactions were due to system failures, such as the misreading of handwritten prescriptions. Subsequent studies sponsored by AHRQ have focused on the detection of medical errors, investigation of diagnostic inaccuracies, the relationship between nurse staffing and adverse events, computerized adverse drug event monitoring, and computer-assisted decisionmaking tools to reduce the potential for errors and improve safety.

In FY 2001, AHRQ invested $50 million in 94 new research grants, contracts, and other projects to reduce medical errors and improve patient safety. This effort represents the Federal government's largest single investment in research on medical errors. These projects will address key unanswered questions about when and how errors occur and provide science-based information on what patients, clinicians, hospital leaders, policymakers, and others can do to make the health care system safer. The results of this research will identify improvement strategies that work in hospitals, doctors' offices, nursing homes, and other health care settings across the Nation. AHRQ's $50 million investment is the first phase of a multi-year effort.

Examples of funded projects in the six major categories of AHRQ's FY 2001 patient safety initiative follow.

- **Collecting and reporting medical errors data.** For example, State health officials in New York and Massachusetts will examine how to improve State-mandated reporting of errors. A project at Harvard Pilgrim Healthcare will evaluate data collected from more than 16,000 primary care physicians participating in 10 of the Nation's leading HMOs to identify medication errors and test ways to prevent them.

- **Using computers and information technology to prevent medical errors.** Researchers at the University of Alabama at Birmingham and Creighton University in Omaha will test whether the use of hand-held computers with decision support systems can reduce medical errors in primary care clinics. At Montefiore Medical Center in New York City, researchers will use computer simulation tools to train surgery residents and to identify, quantify, and analyze errors and "near misses."

- **Working conditions and patient safety.** Researchers will examine how staffing, fatigue, stress, sleep deprivation, organizational culture, shift work, and other factors can lead to errors. For example, researchers at the University of California, San Francisco, will assess the relationship between daily changes in the working conditions in hospitals—including nurse staffing ratios, workload, and skill mix—and medical errors.

- **Innovative approaches to improving patient safety.** One project involves creation of a Center of Excellence in patient Safety Research at the University of Texas in Houston that will apply lessons learned from crew resource management in aviation to build stronger team work in health care. Another project at the University of Chicago will examine how to improve communication and other aspects of team work.

- **Disseminating research results.** Several large health care provider organizations—including the American Hospital Association's Hospital Research and Educational Trust, the American College of Physicians-American Society of Internal Medicine, the American College of Surgeons, and the National Patient Safety Foundation—will partner with AHRQ to disseminate results from patient safety research and test the effectiveness of innovative educational strategies for clinicians. The goal is to better equip health care providers to deliver safe patient care. Another project will study ways of sharing information modeled on hospital and medical school "morbidity and mortality" conferences.

- **Other patient safety initiatives.** These include activities to expand the evidence base on what works and doesn't work in improving safety; meetings of State and local officials to advance local and regional patient safety efforts; funding for small businesses to explore new products to help improve safety; and other initiatives.

Working Conditions and Quality of Care

Increasing our understanding of how working conditions affect health care workers, the risks for errors, and the quality of services provided to patients is of major importance to the health care industry. Recent efforts to reduce costs and streamline the delivery of care have led to significant changes in the health care workplace. The experiences of other industries demonstrate that differences in the equipment and physical characteristics of the workspace, changes in work responsibility and process, and differences in staffing levels can affect the quality of the products or services provided. For example, research on working conditions in the aviation industry has provided evidence of the relationship between aviation safety and work hours, including the effect of factors such as fatigue, lack of sleep, and shift work.

Despite the importance of these factors, there has been scant research focused on the importance of the quality of the workplace environment—not only for worker satisfaction, worker health, and the avoidance of disability, but also for the quality and productivity of the work performed. Workplace factors, including the way work is organized and staffed, may pose a threat, not only to the health and well-being of workers, but also to the quality of care they provide to patients and the safety of the patients.

Working conditions — The characteristics of the health care workplace and workforce, including the physical environment, workflow design, staffing, and organizational culture.

Health care workers — Workers, including physicians, nurses, pharmacists, physician assistants, nursing assistants, and emergency medical technicians who provide direct care to patients in health care settings such as hospitals, ambulatory care settings, and nursing homes.

In FY 2001, AHRQ funded 30 projects that will examine the effects of working conditions on health care workers' ability to provide safe, high-quality care in ambulatory, inpatient (both hospital and long-term care institutions), and home care settings. Examples of the critical issues to be addressed include:

- Effects of extended work hours, sleep deprivation and fatigue, and stress on residents and nurses working in hospital-based settings.

- Relationship between working conditions—such as nurse to patient ratios, workload, and skill mix—and the occurrence or near occurrence of medical errors or adverse events.

37

- Impact of workplace characteristics, organizational culture, and teamwork on the safety, quality, and outcomes of care in inpatient settings, specifically intensive care units and surgical settings.

- Relationship between nursing home working conditions—such as staffing levels, job design, and job satisfaction—and worker outcomes, patient outcomes, and quality of care.

- Impact of financial incentives and the work environment on the quality of care in both ambulatory and inpatient settings.

- Effects of employee training, satisfaction, and understanding of patient safety on patient outcomes and quality of care.

Helping Patients and Consumers Use Quality Information

Americans are demanding greater value and quality in their health care. In today's rapidly changing health care environment, consumers need solid, reliable information to help them choose among health care plans, practitioners, and facilities. They also need information to help them participate more actively and effectively in their personal health care decisions. AHRQ is playing a unique role in providing the information consumers want and need to help them get the best possible health care.

Consumer Assessment of Health Plans

The Consumer Assessment of Health Plans Study (CAHPS®) is an easy-to-use kit of survey and reporting tools that provide reliable information to help consumers and purchasers assess and choose among health plans. Some recent CAHPS accomplishments include:

- AHRQ and the Centers for Medicare & Medicaid Services (CMS) collaborated with the CAHPS consortium to develop a Medicare CAHPS Disenrollee Survey of beneficiaries enrolled in managed care plans that was fielded by CMS. Answers to the survey allow researchers to distinguish disenrollment decisions related to quality (e.g., limited access to specialists) from those that are unrelated to quality (e.g., enrollee moving out of the plan service area).

- Working in collaboration with the California Health Care Foundation and the Pacific Group on Health, the CAHPS team has developed a version of CAHPS to assess care given at the group practice level. This activity is in response to strong consumer interest in the ability of physicians in group practices to provide high-quality care.

- AHRQ and CMS are collaborating in the development of a CAHPS survey to obtain consumers' assessments of health care and services received in nursing homes. Survey development and sampling and data collection procedures were completed in FY 2001. Additional testing will be carried out in FY 2002.

Making Quality Count for Patients and Consumers

AHRQ has funded three demonstration projects to enhance the health care systems' ability to provide patients with information on health care quality. Total projected funding for these three projects is $3.4 million. The researchers will develop and test methods and models for developing information on quality for consumer and patient use in health care decisions, as well as evaluate the impact of strategies to provide information about quality to consumers and patients. The newly funded projects are:

- **Information about quality in a randomized evaluation.** This project underway at the University of California, Davis, will identify factors associated with consumers' use of employer-disseminated information on health plan and medical group performance and determine if and how consumers use or do not use such information during open enrollment.

- **Helping elders include quality in health plan choice.** This project, which is underway at Research Triangle Institute, will develop and evaluate an integrated information and decision support strategy for use by employee benefits staff in counseling employees aged 60 to 64 about their Medicare plan options.

- **Quality factors in nursing home choice.** Researchers at the University of Colorado Health Center will develop and evaluate information strategies to help consumers use quality factors in making nursing home choices.

National Healthcare Quality Report

AHRQ is developing the first-ever annual report on the quality of health care in the United States, as called for in the Agency's reauthorization legislation, which became law in 1999. The goal of the report, now in its early design phase and due out in 2003, is to provide a clear, easily understood picture of the quality of health care in America. The development of a national report on health care quality is an important step in improving the quality of the Nation's health care system and

39

addressing the health care needs of priority populations. See "Research on the Health Care of Priority Populations" in this report (page 52) to learn about AHRQ's program priorities and activities focused on women, children, and minorities.

The project is being led by AHRQ in collaboration with the Centers for Disease Control and Prevention's (CDC's) National Center for Health Statistics. An interagency work group will develop the final content and design of the report. Other members of the work group include the Department's Office of the Assistant Secretary for Planning and Evaluation, CDC, the Centers for Medicare & Medicaid Services, the National Institutes of Health, and the Substance Abuse and Mental Health Services Administration.

As of FY 2001, work on the National Healthcare Quality Report (NHQR) is proceeding as follows:

- A 14-member Institute of Medicine (IOM) committee of leading experts in quality and quality measurement was formed and recommended that the NHQR quality monitoring system be based on a conceptual framework that addresses both dimensions of patient care (e.g., safety, effectiveness, patient centeredness, timeliness, equity) and patient needs (e.g., staying healthy, getting better, living with illness, coping with end-of-life issues).

- AHRQ initiated a call to relevant Federal agencies to identify candidate measures to fill in the conceptual framework. The IOM issued a complementary call for measures to the private sector. Over 400 measures were submitted. An interagency workgroup is evaluating the candidate measures for inclusion in the first report, using criteria suggested by the IOM (e.g., importance, scientific soundness, feasibility).

- AHRQ is identifying and modifying existing data sources to support the NHQR. For example, AHRQ is enhancing its Medical Expenditure Panel Survey (MEPS) by increasing the size and geographic dispersion of the sample and adding quality-related content. AHRQ also has begun a project to look at private-sector data sources, which likely will take on added importance in the future.

- AHRQ is conducting market research to identify the needs of potential audiences for the report and to develop a report design that will meet those needs. We also have begun a project to review existing report systems to help in the development of the NHQR. Future plans include the creation of a Web-based product that will allow users to narrow the focus from national data to get detail on quality performance measures for population subgroups and geographic areas (e.g., regions, States).

National Healthcare Disparities Report

AHRQ is also developing the first-ever report on prevailing disparities in health care delivery in the United States. A large and consistent body of research, much of it funded by AHRQ, has demonstrated persistent disparities in health care quality and access associated with race, ethnicity, socioeconomic position, sex, age, and place of residence. For example, a recent study of Medicare patients revealed that black patients with congestive heart failure or pneumonia received poorer quality care than whites. Further, these differences are associated with greater mortality among black patients.

The Agency's reauthorization legislation, which became law in late 1999, directed AHRQ to develop a report, beginning with fiscal year 2003, on prevailing disparities in health care delivery as they relate to racial factors and socioeconomic factors in priority populations. AHRQ's priority populations include rural, inner-city, low-income groups, minority groups, women, children, the elderly, and individuals with special health care needs. The National Healthcare Disparities Report (NHDR) will serve as a companion document to the National Healthcare Quality Report, providing greater depth and insights into differences in health care quality for priority populations. This report will be an unprecedented effort to present a comprehensive picture of prevailing disparities in health care in the United States, and it will identify opportunities for improving care for priority populations. The report also will provide a benchmark for evaluating the success of programs to reduce disparities in health care.

The project is being led by AHRQ and will involve collaboration with multiple components of the Department of Health and Human Services. As of FY 2001, work on the NHDR is proceeding as follows:

- A 14-member Institute of Medicine (IOM) committee of leading experts in quality measurement, access to care, and disparities in care was formed to inform the framework and content of the NHDR. Building on prior IOM work done for the NHQR, the committee will make recommendations regarding the linkage of the two reports. The IOM also will provide a forum for public input and comment into the design of the NHDR.

41

- Modifications to the Medical Expenditure Panel Survey (MEPS) have been made to allow assessment of quality for priority populations.

- In conjunction with work conducted for the NHQR, AHRQ is conducting market research to identify the needs of potential audiences for the disparities report and to inform the design and format of the report itself.

Goal 3 – Costs, Use, and Access to Health Care

Addressing Challenges to Care

Adequate access to health care services continues to be a challenge for many Americans, particularly those who are poor, uninsured, minorities, rural residents, disabled individuals, and members of other priority populations. Also, continuing changes in the organization and financing of care have raised new questions about access to a range of health services, including emergency and specialty care. At the same time, examples of inappropriate care—including overuse and misuse of services—continue to be identified. Through ongoing development of nationally representative and more specialized databases, the production of public use data products, and research and analyses conducted by AHRQ researchers and AHRQ-funded researchers outside the Agency, we continue to address critical policy issues pertaining to the cost of health care, use of health care services, and access to care.

Examples of findings from recent AHRQ-funded research on health care costs, use of services, and access to care include:

- In many cases, women who have mild to moderate pelvic inflammatory disease (PID) can be successfully treated as outpatients, which would result in substantial cost savings. PID affects more than 1 million U.S. women each year, with annual estimated direct and indirect costs of more than $4 billion. A recent study of more than 800 women with clinical signs and symptoms of mild-to-moderate PID found no apparent differences in rates of pregnancy, infertility, chronic pelvic pain, ectopic pregnancy, or tubal occlusion among women who were hospitalized and those treated as outpatients.

- Hospital mergers may produce lower savings (expenses and revenues per admission) than previously estimated. Researchers examined changes in costs and prices for nearly 1,800 short-term hospitals from 1989 to 1997. They separated nonmerging hospitals into two groups: those that were rivals of the merging hospitals and those that were not competitors. When they compared merging hospitals in high HMO-penetration markets with their nonmerging rivals, the researchers found that the former group's average cost savings were only a modest 2.3 percentage points. Also, the average price growth of merging hospitals in high HMO-penetration markets was almost identical to that of

43

their competitors. On the other hand, the researchers found that mergers in low HMO-penetration markets appear to produce greater cost and price savings for the merging hospitals.

- Increasing AIDS drug assistance program benefits may reduce States' medical expenditures for HIV care. According to this study, if all States that have AIDS drug assistance programs with restricted access to protease inhibitors were to relax those restrictions, their costs would decline because hospital inpatient expenditures would decrease. Also, increasing access to protease inhibitors would reduce a State's total drug expenditures for public beneficiaries with HIV by lowering their need for prescription medicines to fight opportunistic

---

BRIC Research on Health Care Costs

The Building Research Infrastructure and Capacity (BRIC) program launched by AHRQ in FY 2001 provided six awards involving institutions in nine States, including Idaho, Kentucky, Louisiana, Mississippi, Montana, Nevada, New Jersey, Utah, and Wyoming. Many of the projects support the development of partnerships between State agencies and universities to develop data systems useful in evaluating the effects of various programs on the cost and financing of health services. For example:

- **Rutgers Center for Health Services Research.** This grant will enhance a partnership between the State University of New Jersey and State officials to develop and link State health data for use in addressing an array of health services research issues. Investigators will begin by examining the effectiveness of an innovative certificate-of-need strategy to improve access and reduce disparities in cardiac catheterization.

- **Intermountain BRIC Consortium.** This project with the National Association of Health Data Organizations focuses on improving and linking State hospital discharge data with clinical data sets in Intermountain States to assess the economic consequences of policies that influence competition in health care markets.

- **Mississippi Building Research Infrastructure and Capacity.** These researchers will examine the costs and use of health services in order to improve the delivery of primary care to rural, low-income populations in the Mississippi Delta area. The researchers will identify gaps in services and how these gaps could be addressed through telemedicine and increasing the efficiency of mobile care units.

infections. The researchers warn, however, that expanding these State programs would likely increase costs per public beneficiary.

- Coronary angiography is underused for both Medicare managed care and fee-for-service heart attack patients. This study showed that Medicare patients enrolled in managed care plans are significantly less likely than those with traditional Medicare fee-for-service coverage to receive needed coronary angiography following a heart attack, a potentially life-saving procedure. These findings also bear out the underuse of the procedure in general; 66 percent of class I patients in Medicare managed care did not receive the procedure, compared with 54 percent of class I Medicare enrollees with fee-for-service coverage. Class I patients are those judged most in need of the procedure according to American College of Cardiology and American Heart Association guidelines.

Medical Expenditure Panel Survey

AHRQ's Medical Expenditure Panel Survey (MEPS) provides highly detailed information on how Americans use and pay for health care. In addition to the core MEPS survey of households, it includes surveys of medical providers and establishments to supplement the data provided by household respondents on medical expenditures and health insurance coverage. The design of the MEPS survey permits both person-based and family-level estimates. The scope and depth of this data collection effort reflect the needs of government agencies, legislative bodies, and health professionals for comprehensive national estimates for use in the formulation and analysis of national health policies.

The MEPS collects data on the specific health services that Americans use, how frequently they use them, the cost of these services, and how they are paid for, as well as data on the cost, scope, and breadth of private health insurance held by and available to the U.S. population. This ongoing survey of about 15,000 households each year provides estimates for the country as a whole and for important priority populations. MEPS is unparalleled for the degree of detail in its data and its ability to link health service use, medical expenditures, and health insurance data to the demographic, employment, economic, health status, and other characteristics of survey respondents. Moreover, the MEPS provides a foundation for estimating the impact of changes affecting access to insurance or medical care on economic groups or special populations of interest, such as the poor, the elderly, veterans, the uninsured, and racial and ethnic minorities.

- **Databases.** MEPS produces a number of analytical databases and, consistent with privacy policy, releases a number of databases to the public. These

45

46

How MEPS data are used:

- In the public sector (e.g., Office of Management and Budget, Medicare Payment Advisory Commission, and Treasury Department): Government agencies and Congress rely on MEPS data to evaluate health reform policies, the effects of tax code changes on health expenditures and tax revenue, and proposed changes in government health programs such as Medicare.

- In the private sector (e.g., RAND, Heritage Foundation, and the Urban Institute): Businesses, foundations, and academic institutions use these data to develop economic projections.

- For research: These data represent a major resource for the health services research community at large. In the past year, data on premium costs from the MEPS Insurance Component have been used by the Bureau of Economic Analysis to produce estimates of the gross domestic product (GDP) for the Nation.

---

databases include demographic, health care use, access, expense, and insurance coverage information for all survey participants. Additional files detailing conditions, the specific content of health care events, and employment of household respondents also are made available to the public.

- **Printed data.** In addition to providing databases for research use, AHRQ publishes MEPS data in tabular form on a range of topics. For example, each year AHRQ releases hundreds of tables on the health insurance coverage offered by employers. The data are available for the Nation as a whole, for important economic sectors, and for many States.

- **Web site.** To maximize the use of this important investment, AHRQ has developed a Web site specific to the MEPS. This Web site rapidly disseminates databases and other products to the research community and quickly responds to inquiries from MEPS data users. In FY 2001, AHRQ was responding to more than 100 inquiries made through the Web site each month.

- **Training.** To develop a cadre of sophisticated MEPS users outside of AHRQ, the Agency conducts a series of workshops, which range in length from a few hours to several days. They provide orientation to the policymaker and researcher about the range of questions that MEPS can answer and how the data can be properly used.

- **Data Center.** AHRQ's Center for Cost and Financing Studies operates a Data Center to facilitate access to and use of MEPS data and answer questions from users.

MEPS Products and Key Findings

Key findings, 2000:

- In the first half of 2000, about 16 percent of the U.S. civilian noninstitutionalized population was uninsured.

- Among those under age 65, Hispanics accounted for about 25 percent of the uninsured population in 2000, even though they represented only about 13 percent of the overall population for this age group.

Key findings, 1999

- Among adults under age 65, married people were more likely to have health insurance.

- About 82 percent of Americans under age 65 had public or private insurance coverage.

Key findings, 1998:

- More than 50 percent of elderly Americans had private insurance, but more than 40 percent had only public coverage (Medicare with or without Medicaid).

- Less than half of all Hispanic Americans and about half of black Americans were covered by private health insurance, compared with three-quarters of whites.

Key findings, 1997:

- More than one-third of young adults (aged 19-24) were uninsured in 1997.

- Among all racial/ethnic groups, Hispanic males were the most likely to be uninsured; nearly 37 percent lacked coverage.

- During the first half of 1997, almost 30 percent of children under age 4, 25 percent of those ages 4-6, and about 20 percent of children ages 7-12 had only public insurance coverage.

MEPS Household Component[1]

Key findings, 1996:

- Inpatient hospital care accounts for nearly $4 of very $10 spent on health care.

- Prescription medicines account for about 12 percent of total expenditures.

- Almost 53 percent of children covered by Medicaid have a parent that works.

- Only about 43 percent of the population received dental care in 1996.

- Nearly 32 percent of Hispanics and 21 percent of blacks were insured in 1998, compared with only 12 percent of whites.

[1]Full-year data have been released for 1996-1998; partial-year data have been released for 1999-2000.

continued

MEPS Insurance Component[2]

Key findings:

- The average health insurance premium in 1996 was $1,997 for single coverage and $4,953 for a family; in 1999, the average premiums were $2,325 (single) and $6,058 (family).

- Over the period 1996-1999, rates of contribution for employers and employees have remained the same.

- In every State, establishments in large firms (50 or more employees) were more likely to offer health insurance than those in small firms (less than 50 employees).

- For both single and family plans, more workers were covered by mixed-provider (PPO-type) plans than were covered by any-provider (conventional indemnity-type) plans or exclusive-provider plans (like HMOs). Enrollment rates in mixed-provider plans increased over the 1996-1999 period.

- About 70 percent of U.S. establishments that offer health insurance offer only one plan; employers in Hawaii and California are most likely to offer their employees a choice of plans.

[2] Data are available for 1996-1999.

Healthcare Cost and Utilization Project

The unprecedented volume and pace of change in the U.S. health care system, and the fact that changes are not occurring uniformly across the country, require a new information standard. We at AHRQ have long recognized the need for scientifically sound, standardized databases and tools for using them, as well as the need to make these resources available at the national, regional, and State levels.

State Inpatient Databases (SID). The SID comprise non-Federal hospital discharge data from the participating States (see below), which represent about 67 percent of the over 22 million inpatient discharge abstracts in the United States.

Arizona*	Georgia	Maine	New Jersey*
Tennessee	California*	Hawaii	Maryland*
New York*	Utah*	Colorado*	Illinois
Massachusetts*	Oregon*	Virginia	Connecticut
Iowa*	Michigan	Pennsylvania	Washington*
Florida*	Kansas	Missouri	Wisconsin*
South Carolina*			

*Participants in AHRQ's designated central distributor or single point of contact to facilitate access to their databases.

The Healthcare Cost and Utilization Project is one of many ways in which AHRQ is addressing this need.

HCUP is a Federal-State-industry partnership to build a standardized, multi-State health data system. This long-standing partnership has built and continues to develop and expand a family of administrative databases and powerful, user-friendly software to enhance the use of administrative data. Included in HCUP is hospital discharge information from State-specific hospital and ambulatory surgery databases, as well as a national sample of discharges from community hospitals. HCUP data are used at all levels to inform decisionmaking. HCUP continues to be a very valuable resource in light of recent findings that about 40 percent of personal health care expenditures in the United States go towards hospital care—making it the most expensive component of the health care sector.

> **Nationwide Inpatient Sample (NIS)** is the largest all-payer inpatient database in the United States. It provides information on about 7 million inpatient discharges from about 1,000 hospitals, including data from 1988-1999. According to NIS data:
>
> - About 135,000 hospital stays a year for treatment of depression, and alcohol- and substance-related mental disorders are not covered by either private insurance or public insurance programs such as Medicare and Medicaid
>
> - Childbirth is the leading type of hospital care not covered by private insurance or public coverage. About 5 percent of all hospitalizations for childbirth—roughly 191,000 hospital stays a year—are uninsured.
>
> - Two chronic diseases, which if appropriately treated in primary care practices do not ordinarily result in hospitalization, also are among the top 10 types of uninsured inpatient care—asthma and diabetes. Together they account for 65,000 hospital admissions a year.

FY 2001 accomplishments include increasing the number of States participating in HCUP; now half (25) of all States are HCUP partners, an increase of roughly 15 percent over the previous fiscal year. New State partners were selected based on the diversity—in terms of geographic representation and population ethnicity—they bring to the project, along with data quality performance and their ability to facilitate timely processing of data.

AHRQ also expanded HCUP beyond inpatient hospital settings to include hospital-based State ambulatory surgery databases (SASD). The number of States participating in the SASD increased from 9 in FY 2000 to 13 in FY 2001.

49

> **State Ambulatory Surgery Databases (SASD)** include data on surgeries performed on the same day in which patients are admitted and released from hospital-affiliated ambulatory surgery sites.
>
> | | | |
> |---|---|---|
> | Colorado* | Maryland* | Pennsylvania |
> | Wisconsin | Connecticut | Missouri |
> | South Carolina | Florida | New Jersey* |
> | Tennessee | Maine | New York* |
> | Utah | | |
>
> *Participates in AHRQ's designated central distributor or single point of contact to facilitate access to their databases.

Additionally, a pilot of emergency department databases was expanded from one to five States. The State Emergency Department Databases (SEDD) capture hospital-affiliated emergency department encounters from data organizations in participating States.

AHRQ recently announced the availability of the Kids' Inpatient Database (KID), the first comprehensive research database exclusively concerned with inpatient care of children and adolescents in the Nation's community hospitals. The KID is the only dataset on hospital use, outcomes, and charges for children age 18 and younger, including newborns, regardless of whether they are privately insured, receive public assistance, or have no health insurance. The KID contains national estimates for 6.7 million pediatric discharges and data on various hospital characteristics such as region, location (urban/rural), size, ownership, and pediatric hospital status.

During the past year AHRQ began a multifaceted effort to make HCUP data more accessible to researchers and other interested users. A centerpiece of this effort is HCUPnet, a free, interactive, menu-driven online service that allows easy access to national statistics and trends and selected State statistics about hospital stays.

HCUPnet answers questions about conditions treated and procedures performed in hospitals for the population as a whole, as well as for subsets of the population such as children and the elderly. In addition, 10 States have agreed to include their data in HCUPnet. About 4,000 visits are logged each month on HCUPnet, which can be found at www.ahrp.gov/data/hcup/hcupnet.htm.

A second key component of our effort to facilitate researchers' access to HCUP data is the creation of a central distribution center for the State-level databases. Now researchers can go one-stop shopping instead of contacting each State on an individual basis.

Data from HCUP have been used to produce reports that answer questions on reasons Americans are hospitalized, how long they stay in the hospital, the procedures they undergo, how specific conditions are treated in hospitals, and the resulting outcomes. In FY 2001, AHRQ launched an HCUP factbook series that is disseminated in print and through the AHRQ Web site. These factbooks were downloaded nearly 40,000 times in the first 6 months after they were posted on the Agency's Web site. Examples of information provided in the HCUP factbooks include:

- The top five reasons for hospital admission are births, coronary arteriosclerosis, pneumonia, congestive heart failure, and heart attack.

- Organ transplantation is associated with some of the longest and most expensive hospital stays.

- Over one-third of all hospital admissions are through the emergency department.

- The average charge for a hospital stay is over $110,000, and the average length of hospital stay is about 5 days.

- Medicare and Medicaid are billed for about 54 percent of all hospital stays.

Research on the Health of Priority Populations

Health Care for Minorities, Women, and Children

The overall health of the American people has improved over the last several decades, but not all Americans have shared equally in these improvements. Among nonelderly adults, for example, 17 percent of Hispanic and 16 percent of black Americans report their health status as only fair or poor, compared with 10 percent of white Americans. How much do differences in the quality and types of health care services that people receive contribute to disparities in health? What strategies can we employ to overcome these differences in care? Answers to these and many other related questions are being sought through AHRQ-sponsored research.

AHRQ is preparing a national report on health care quality to be published for the first time in FY 2003. It will address many health care issues that are particularly important to vulnerable populations. See page 39 of this report for more information on the national report on health care quality.

Disparities in health care and outcomes persist despite improvements in health for the Nation as a whole. AHRQ research found that race and ethnicity influence a patient's chance of receiving many specific procedures and treatments. Of nine hospital procedures investigated in one study, five were significantly less common among black patients than white patients; three of the five procedures also were less common among Hispanics, and two were less common among Asian Americans. Other AHRQ-supported studies have revealed other disparities in patient care, including the following examples.

- Blacks are 13 percent less likely to undergo coronary angioplasty and one-third less likely to undergo bypass surgery than whites.

- Among preschool children hospitalized for asthma, only 7 percent of black and 2 percent of Hispanic children, compared with 21 percent of white children, are prescribed routine medications to prevent future asthma-related hospitalizations.

- The length of time between an abnormal screening mammogram and the followup diagnostic test to determine whether a woman has breast cancer is more than twice as long for Asian American, black, and Hispanic women as it is for white women.

- Blacks with HIV are less likely than other people with HIV to be on antiretroviral therapy, to receive preventive medicine for pneumonia, or to be given protease inhibitors.

- Black, Asian American, and Hispanic residents of nursing homes are far less likely than white residents to have sensory and communication aids, such as glasses and hearing aids.

We ensure that the Agency's research emphasizes the needs of priority populations who generally are underserved by the health care system and underrepresented in research. In FY 2001, the Agency began assembling an office dedicated to research on priority populations that will focus on children, women, and minorities, the elderly and aging population, people with disabilities and/or chronic diseases, people who are terminally ill, people living in the inner city, rural residents, and low-income individuals and families.

Other AHRQ efforts undertaken in this area in 2001 include:

- **Established nine Excellence Centers to Eliminate Ethnic/Racial Disparities (EXCEED).** This 5-year effort will bring together teams of new and experienced investigators to analyze the factors that contribute to ethnic and racial inequities in health care and identify practical tools and strategies to eliminate the disparities.

- **Began data development required to produce the National Disparities Report.** The report will address trends in health care disparities and compare access, use, and quality of health care services as they relate to race, ethnicity, and socioeconomic factors in priority populations.

- **Expanded the HIV Research Network.** This expansion will allow researchers to compare current data on HIV care and examine whether disparities in care among groups are being addressed, as well as identify any new patterns in treatment. The Network receives data from a large number of HIV providers around the Nation in order to provide valid and reliable information about the determinants of resource use by people with HIV disease. See page 62 for more information on the HIV Research Network.

- **Developed numerous Spanish-language publications.** These materials support patient decisionmaking—for example, the Consumer Assessment of Health Plans Study (CAHPS®), which assesses consumers' satisfaction with their health care and helps them select among health plans, and booklets from the Put Prevention Into Practice program that people can use to track whether they or their children have received recommended preventive services.

53

Minority Health

AHRQ and its predecessor agencies (NCHSR and AHCPR) have been involved in research on minority health issues for more than three decades. AHRQ's investments in minority health services research have resulted in numerous findings that are helping to shed light on the disparities experienced by racial and ethnic minorities and expand what is known about the reasons for those disparities.

In FY 2001, AHRQ funded a number of grants with a major emphasis on minority health. This effort includes the launch of the Minority Research Infrastructure Support Program (M-RISP), a training program to increase the number of minority health services researchers and to expand the Nation's health workforce to be more diverse and representative of the racial and ethnic populations in America.

Examples of findings from recent AHRQ supported research follow.

- About one black woman in four over 55 years of age has diabetes, which is nearly twice the rate of diabetes among white women. Hispanic women are almost twice as likely to have diabetes as non-Hispanic women of similar ages.

- Although breast cancer mortality declined 5.6 percent between 1990 and 1994, the decline was much greater among white women at 6.1 percent than among black women at 1 percent.

- Black Medicare beneficiaries are far less likely than white beneficiaries to receive flu shots, regardless of whether they are enrolled in a managed care or fee-for service health plan—68 percent of whites versus 46 percent of blacks received flu shots.

- Hispanics in their 50s are much less likely than same-age whites or blacks to take medication to control high blood pressure.

Women's Health

AHRQ supports research that improves the quality, outcomes, and access to effective health care for women. One specific focus of the women's health program is research that enhances active life expectancy for older women. Although women in the United States are living longer than ever before, on average they experience 3.1 years of disability at the end of life—that is, they experience a decreased ability to function independently due to chronic illnesses. Today, the chronic conditions of heart disease, cancer, and stroke account for 63 percent of deaths among American women, and heart disease causes more than one-third of these deaths. AHRQ currently is supporting development of an unprecedented evidence report to clarify which diagnostic and therapeutic interventions for heart disease are most effective for women, as well as studies that evaluate strategies to improve functional outcomes for older women.

A second major focus for AHRQ's women's health research consists of studies to improve the response of health care organizations and clinicians to victims of domestic violence, the second leading cause of injuries and death among women of childbearing age. Working closely with the HHS's Office of Women's Health and private-sector organizations, AHRQ convened a meeting of experts to develop a health services research agenda focused on the health care consequences of domestic violence. This agenda resulted in a targeted research initiative consisting of projects, conducted in a broad array of practice settings, to improve detection and management of women who experience domestic violence. AHRQ hosted a Senior Scholar-in-Residence to work on projects to provide scientific information on the cost, quality, and outcomes of domestic violence intervention programs available to victims in health care settings. The women will be followed over time to identify interventions that improve the health and safety of victims, predict and improve health care use, prevent and reduce the occurrence of domestic violence, and develop better techniques to identify women at risk for domestic violence.

To support the next generation of researchers, AHRQ is collaborating with the National Institutes of Health, Office of Research on Women's Health, in the Building Interdisciplinary Research Careers in Women's Health program (BIRCWH) to include a health services research component in support of the interdisciplinary focus of the programs to be developed.

Selected examples of recent findings from AHRQ-supported studies include:

- The incidence of coronary heart disease in women has increased over the past decade, yet evidence suggests that women typically receive fewer high-technology cardiac procedures than men. Before age 75, women are more likely than men to die in the hospital after a heart attack.

- ER doctors misdiagnose about 2 percent of patients with heart attack or stable angina because they do not have chest pain or other symptoms typically associated with heart attack. When these patients are mistakenly sent home from the ER, they are twice as likely to die from their heart problems as similar patients who are admitted to the hospital.

- Blacks and women are significantly less likely to be referred for cardiac catheterization than whites and men.

Children's Health

Improving outcomes, quality, and access to health care for America's 70 million children and adolescents is a critical goal of health services research and central to the mission of AHRQ. Understanding what's needed to improve health care delivery for children and adolescents requires a special research focus.

Because children are growing and developing, their health care needs and resource use differ from adults. Unlike adults, they usually are dependent on others for access to care and determinations about the quality of care they receive. Several AHRQ-funded studies on children's health have shown the importance of experience in caring for children.

AHRQ's work helps to fill the major gap that exists in evidence-based information on the health care needs of children and adolescents. Such information is essential to appropriately guide clinical and policy decisions. The need for this information has become particularly critical since the implementation of the State Child Health Insurance Program (SCHIP).

The Child Health Insurance Research Initiative (CHIRI), cofunded by AHRQ, the David and Lucile Packard Foundation, and the Health Resources Services Administration (HRSA), is a 3-year research program designed to identify which health insurance and delivery features work best for low-income children, particularly minority children and those with special health care needs. Results from the nine CHIRI™ projects will aid in understanding how to improve health care for vulnerable children, including children who remain uninsured, and how to improve the institutions that serve them. Researchers and funders participate in a collaborative process to strengthen individual studies and increase the generalizability of results, making it possible for CHIRI™ findings to be applied across locations, populations, and insurance design and organizational delivery system features.

CHIRI™ researchers work closely with local and national policymakers to ensure that the projects generate information that is useful and timely for decisionmakers. For example:

In Kansas, CHIRI™ researchers found that many enrollees in the Kansas SCHIP had previously been recipients of Medicaid, and a significant proportion subsequently transferred from SCHIP to Medicaid. In addition, the researchers found that 23 percent of Kansas families who have a child in SCHIP also have a child in Medicaid. These findings were shared with State legislators and administrators of Kansas' public insurance programs and contributed to a decision to integrate Kansas Medicaid and SCHIP under a single delivery system.

- The method used by SCHIP programs to periodically redetermine the eligibility of enrollees has an impact on continuity of coverage. State eligibility redetermination requirements for SCHIP enrollees generated large disenrollments in three of four States that were studied, though up to one-quarter of children returned within 2 months. In the fourth State, a passive reenrollment policy eliminated excess disenrollment at the point of eligibility redetermination.

To address the scarcity of quality measures for children, AHRQ is supporting the development, testing, and implementation of the Pediatric Quality of Life measures. Also, the National Committee for Quality Assurance for HEDIS adopted the children's component of AHRQ's Consumer Assessment of Health Plan Study (CAHPS) survey—the first time a health-plan-oriented survey of children was administered nationwide.

In FY 2001, AHRQ supported child-relevant studies focused on outcomes, quality and patient safety, and cost, use, and access. Researchers involved in these studies are working to:

- Develop the first comprehensive analysis of the management of suspected child abuse in primary care practices.

- Develop and evaluate a computerized laptop system for use in the examining room of primary care practices as an extension of an existing in-house prescribing system to improve the care of children with attention-deficit/hyperactivity disorder.

- Investigate the impact of having a child with asthma and the burden this condition causes on the family's resources (e.g., finances, the parents' time and availability for care, and access and barriers to health care).

- Identify strategies to improve ambulatory antibiotic prescribing practices. For example, the researchers will measure and assess changes in antibiotic prescription rates for sore throat in children and bronchitis in adults using managed care and Medicaid data from physicians' practices.

- Focus on children with special health care needs to identify those factors parents consider when choosing a managed care plan, identify difficulties children have in accessing care, and assess several quality of care indicators, such as receipt of preventive services (e.g., immunizations), dental care, referrals to specialists, appropriateness of medication use, hospitalizations for ambulatory care-sensitive conditions, and continuity of care.

Recent findings from AHRQ-supported child health research:

- Children who have chronic conditions and are enrolled in Medicaid receive most of their care from generalist physicians rather than specialists.

- The P3C, a new measure of parents' perceptions of primary care quality, was developed by AHRQ-supported researchers and found to be practical, reliable, and valid. The measure was tested in English, Spanish, Vietnamese, and Tagalog.

- Therapies and outcomes for pediatric head trauma patients vary across pediatric ICUs. Large randomized, controlled trials are needed to determine whether increased use of seizure medications or other therapies could improve outcomes.

- Children in Medicaid managed care receive care equal to that of privately insured children in terms of access to care, use of services, and satisfaction with care.

- Children are vaccinated later in the practices of providers who do not receive free vaccine supplies, those that refer uninsured children to a public vaccine clinic, and providers who over-interpret contraindications to vaccination.

Rapid Cycle Research

Bioterrorism

Prior to the events of September 11, 2001, there was little experience in the United States with bioterrorist incidents. The reality of bioterrorism has focused attention on the need for a strong health infrastructure to coordinate, prepare for, and respond to acts of terrorism, particularly those involving biological or chemical agents.

AHRQ's investment in bioterrorism research draws from the recognition that clinicians, hospitals, and health care systems have essential roles in the public health infrastructure. AHRQ research focuses on the health care of the general population by training clinicians to recognize manifestations of bioterrorism agents and manage patients appropriately, assessing the preparedness of hospitals and health systems to respond to bioterrorism incidents, and helping State and local policymakers respond to bioterrorism.

Examples of products and tools supported by AHRQ that are currently or soon will be available include the following:

- Researchers at the University of Alabama at Birmingham and Research Triangle Institute have developed Web-based training modules to teach health professionals how to address varied biologicat agents. Separate modules exist for ER practitioners, radiologists, pathologists, and infection control specialists. These clinicians can obtain continuing medical education (CME) credit at this site (www.bioterrorism.uab.edu).

- Through collaborations with the University of Maryland, Emory University, the District of Columbia Hospital Association, and Booz-Allen Hamilton, a questionnaire has been developed that can help assess the current level of preparedness of hospitals or health systems and their capacity to respond to bioterrorism attacks.

- In collaboration with the New York City Department of Health and the Mayor's Office of Emergency Management, AHRQ's Integrated Delivery System Research Network based at the Weill Medical College of Cornell University has developed a computer simulation model for city-wide response planning for bioterrorism attacks. This model for mass prevention of disease in the event of a bioterrorism incident will be validated by a live exercise funded by the Department of Justice.

- Researchers at the Children's Hospital of Boston are exploring the feasibility of building decision support models for information systems using linked health care data. These information systems would help to link the public health infrastructure with the clinical care delivery system to speed reporting and enhance rapid dissemination of relevant information. A preliminary product is a literature review that clarifies the potential of Web-based systems for clinicians to obtain timely information and report potential bioterrorism events to public health authorities.

- Researchers at the University of Pittsburgh and Carnegie-Mellon are continuing development of a Real-time Outbreak and Disease Surveillance (RODS) system for bioterrorism events. The purpose of RODS is to provide early warning of infectious disease outbreaks, possibly caused by an act of bioterrorism, so that treatment and control measures can be initiated to protect and save large numbers of people.

- The Science Applications International Corporation (SAIC) in collaboration with Johns Hopkins University, George Washington University, and the Joint Commission on Accreditation of Healthcare Organizations (JCAHO) has completed extensive work on assessing and recommending improvement in the linkages between the medical care, public health, and emergency preparedness systems to detect and respond to bioterrorism events.

- AHRQ's User Liaison Program is planning an audio teleconference in January 2002 for State and local health policymakers to inform them of related research findings that could help them assess and strengthen the capacity of the health care system within their jurisdictions to respond to bioterrorism.

- The Primary Care Practice-Based Research Network at the University of Indiana is using a city-wide electronic medical records system as a model for surveillance and detection of potential bioterrorism events across a wide range of health care facilities, including primary care practices, public health clinics, emergency rooms, and hospitals.

Integrated Delivery System Research Network

Improving care practices and collecting evidence about what works and what does not work in our largely private health care system requires use of private-sector data and partnerships between researchers and providers of care. Private-sector databases generally are not accessible to most of the scientific research community. The Integrated Delivery System Research Network (IDSRN), a new model of research developed this past year, links the Nation's top researchers and some of the largest health care systems with AHRQ. In so doing, it enables AHRQ researchers to conduct studies and collect information available only in the private sector to address DHHS' public policy priorities and develop evidence that health system leaders can use to improve care. The IDSRN comprises nine partner organizations that provide care to over 50 million Americans, including privately insured patients, Medicare and Medicaid patients, the uninsured, ethnic and racial minorities, and rural and inner-city residents.

AHRQ funded 16 projects in FY 2001, with timelines that range from 12 to 18 months. Eleven of these projects focus on improving patient safety and working conditions for health care workers, and five focus on reducing disparities in health care delivery. Specifically, the researchers will:

- Examine the extent of variation in performance on HEDIS (Health Plan Employer Data and Information Set) measures for cardiovascular care and diabetes, a cardiac risk factor, by race/ethnicity, socioeconomic status, and sex across, between, and within health plans and evaluate the desirability and feasibility of stratified reporting of quality measures by health plans. In this study, which is now completed, researchers found moderate to large differences in health plan performance on multiple HEDIS measures by race and socioeconomic status, with some plans performing much better for black and low-income enrolles than others. They found that geocoding is a valid methodology for assessing disparities in the absence of data on the race and ethnicity of enrollees.

- Examine ways to improve the care delivered to women, children, minority populations, and patients with limited English proficiency. This will enhance the capacity of health plans and health care delivery systems to identify and address disparities in health care delivery within their populations.

Primary Care Practice-Based Research Networks

Over the past decade, primary care practice-based research networks (PBRNs) have emerged as a promising approach to the scientific study of primary care. These "living laboratories" draw on the experience and insight of practicing clinicians to identify and frame research questions whose answers can improve the practice of primary care.

A PBRN is a group of ambulatory practices devoted principally to the primary care of patients, affiliated with each other (and often with an academic or professional organization) in order to investigate questions related to community-

61

based practice. By linking these questions with rigorous research methods, the PBRN can produce research findings that are immediately relevant to the clinician and more easily translated into everyday practice. In addition, data are readily available on who receives care, how often they receive care, and where care is provided.

AHRQ's overall goal is to improve the capacity of PBRNs to expand the primary care knowledge base, establish mechanisms to ensure that new knowledge is incorporated into actual practice, and make sure its impact is assessed. AHRQ funded 18 networks in FY 2001 through cooperative agreements for infrastructure development and network-defining surveys. All 18 networks will conduct surveys that will provide baseline data on the clinicians enrolled in each network, the services provided, and the characteristics of patients receiving those services.

Many of the networks will also conduct special projects. For example:

- Four of the networks were awarded additional funds to pilot test and evaluate electronic methods of collecting and aggregating practice-derived research data. One of these projects, being conducted within the national network of the American Academy of Family Physicians, will test the use of hand-held computers to improve pneumococcal immunization among adults.

- Two networks were awarded additional funds to assess clinician and patient knowledge and attitudes about protecting the privacy and confidentiality of research data. The network supported by the University of California, San Francisco will, for example, conduct in-depth interviews to learn patient attitudes and perceptions regarding research participation generally, and release of medical record information specifically.

- Two networks were awarded grants that focus on patient safety reporting systems in primary care practice. One of these networks, sponsored by the University of Colorado, will test various patient safety reporting systems in community practices that serve rural, urban, minority, and other underserved populations.

HIV Research Network

Swift changes in treatment regimens resulting from continuous drug therapies are having a profound effect on resource use by people with HIV infection. Medicaid, Medicare, the Department of Veterans Affairs, and the Ryan White CARE Act spend more than $7 billion each year to treat people with HIV disease. Yet, because change is occurring so quickly, data that were collected as recently as

3 years ago do not reflect the current situation and cannot be used reliably for policy and planning purposes.

In 1999, AHRQ joined with the Department's Assistant Secretary for Policy and Evaluation (ASPE), the Substance Abuse and Mental Health Services Administration (SAMHSA), and the Health Resources and Services Administration (HRSA) to establish a pilot HIV data center at the Johns Hopkins School of Medicine. The goal was to collect current information about a large number of individuals who have HIV disease from providers who specialize in HIV care and build a set of associated, publicly available databases about the characteristics of patients and the care they receive. Although the HIV Research Network produces real-time information about access, costs, and quality of care, its databases will not include any patient or provider identifiers.

In 1999, researchers at the data center tested on a small scale the feasibility of transmitting data from HIV caregivers. These included data on patient characteristics, payer data, clinical data, and data on the number of visits and admissions. In the initial phase of this project, the researchers succeeded in enrolling a set of HIV care providers in different regions of the United States and in establishing procedures for transferring data on HIV-related resource use and relevant clinical parameters to the HIV Research Network. Data on over 10,000 HIV-infected patients for calendar year 1999 were transferred to the HIV Research Network.

In FY 2000, the pilot was deemed successful, NIH's Office of AIDS Research joined the collaboration, and efforts were expanded to collect data from 20 to 30 providers who treat at least 20,000 people with HIV disease. Preliminary data analyses indicate that there are serious disparities among people with HIV disease in their ability to receive expensive new drug therapies. Specifically, analyses show:

- Black women covered by Medicaid are less likely than other patients to receive new and expensive drug therapies.

- White patients are more likely than black or Hispanic patients to receive new therapies.

- Medicaid patients are less likely than privately insured patients to receive new drugs.

In FY 2001, based on the promising results from the pilot project, AHRQ initiated a contract to continue the project through FY 2005.

The HIV Research Network provides an ongoing means to collect timely information on resource use associated with HIV disease. It is a cost-effective way to obtain reasonably complete medical and financial information on a large number of HIV-infected patients, thus facilitating research on HIV care among different types of patients. Future plans include enrolling several new pediatric sites to examine access to care for children with HIV, as well as the costs and quality of care they receive. In addition, the HIV Research Network plans to conduct interviews with patients at each site to acquire information about their compliance with medication dosages and their access to mental health and substance abuse services.

User Liaison Program

AHRQ's User Liaison Program (ULP) synthesizes and distributes research findings to local and State policymakers so they can use it to make evidence-based decisions about health care policy. ULP holds small workshops, sponsors audio teleconferences, and distributes other information to provide recent research findings to policymakers on the critical issues confronting them in today's changing health care marketplace. These products are user-driven and user-designed. ULP solicits input from legislators, executive agency staff, and local officials on policy issues where they need information and technical assistance.

In FY 2001, ULP held 18 workshops attended by more than 1,500 health care policymakers representing all States, the District of Columbia, American Samoa, the Virgin Islands, and Guam. Eight of these were national workshops attended by policymakers from around the country, and two workshops were held for specific audiences. In addition, ULP conducted four audio-teleconferences—expanding long-term choices for the elderly, strengthening the health care safety net, the paraprofessional workforce, and health care informatics—that brought training directly to 800 policymakers and other interested parties.

Financial Management

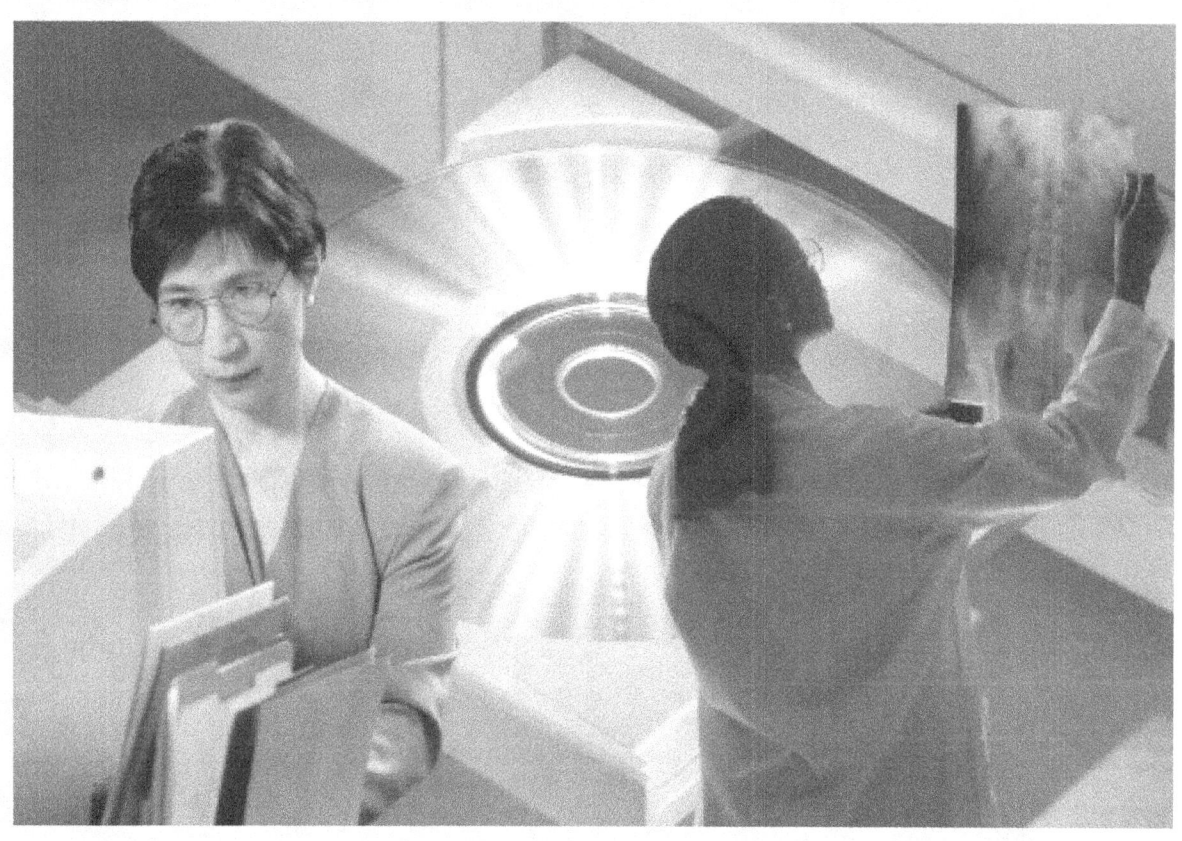

Financial Management Performance

Overview of Financial Performance

The Director, Office of Management (OM) serves as the Chief Financial Officer (CFO), and as such is responsible for overseeing all financial management activities relating to the programs and operation of the Agency. The CFO is accountable for ensuring that the financial management legislation, such as the Chief Financial Officers (CFOs) Act of 1990, the Federal Managers Financial Integrity Act (FMFIA) of 1992, and the Government Management and Reform Act (GMRA) of 1994, are implemented.

The Division of Financial Management, a component of OM, takes the lead in providing services and guidance in all aspects of Agency financial management, including budget formulation and execution, funds control, appropriation legislation, and development of automated financial management systems. AHRQ purchases its fund accounting, financial reporting, debt management, and other related fiscal services from the Program Support Center's (PSC) Division of Financial Operations (DFO) on a fee for service basis. Because the Department prepares audited financial statements for its largest components only, AHRQ financial statements are not audited.

Budgetary Resources

AHRQ receives its funding through an annual discretionary appropriation that includes Federal funds and miscellaneous reimbursements. The reimbursements come from other Federal agencies, usually in the form of expenditure transfers (payments made from one account to another). In addition, AHRQ receives modest funds from Freedom of Information Act fees.

Mechanisms of Support

AHRQ provides financial support to public and private nonprofit entities and individuals through the award of grants, cooperative agreements, contracts, and interagency agreements (IAAs). The grant and cooperative agreement mechanisms are used for activities where there is a public purpose authorized by statute that must be accomplished. The contract mechanism is used when the required product or service is for the direct use or benefit of the Federal government. IAAs

67

AHRQ Appropriations by Funding Source
(Dollars in Millions)

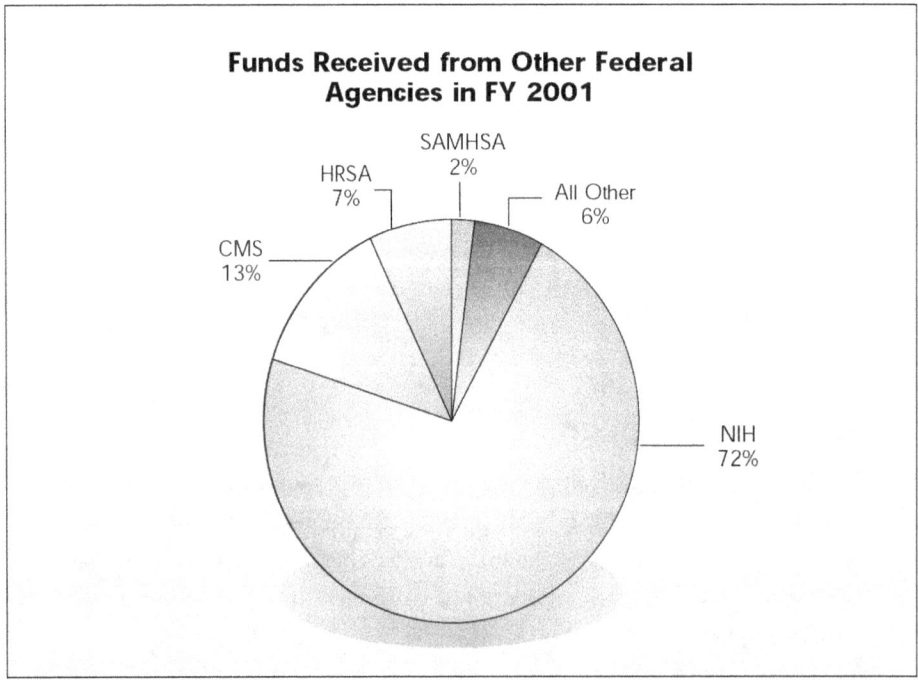

Fiscal Year

☐ Trust Funds ☐ 1% Evaluation ☐ Budget Authority

Excludes Y2K and Bioterrorism Funds

Funds Received from Other Federal Agencies in FY 2001

SAMHSA
2%

HRSA
7%

All Other
6%

CMS
13%

NIH
72%

are used to provide to, purchase from, or exchange goods or services with another federal agency.

Program Announcements (PAs) are employed to invite applications for new or ongoing grant activities of a general nature, and Requests for Applications (RFAs) are used to invite grant applications for a targeted area. In FY 2001, 59 percent of AHRQ grants and cooperative agreements were in response to RFAs, and 41 percent were in response to RFAs, and initiated by individual investigators who developed research proposals within an area of interest to the Agency.

AHRQ also supports small grants that facilitate the initiation of studies for preliminary short-term projects, dissertation grants undertaken as part of an academic program to earn a research doctoral degree, conference grants that complement and promote AHRQ's core research and help the Agency further its mission, and National Research Services Awards (NRSAs) that support predoctoral and postdoctoral trainees through grants to individuals and institutions such as medical schools and universities.

The Agency awards minority supplements to ongoing grants that have at least 2 years of committed support remaining. These supplements are used to train and provide health services research experience to minorities or to support research on minority health issues.

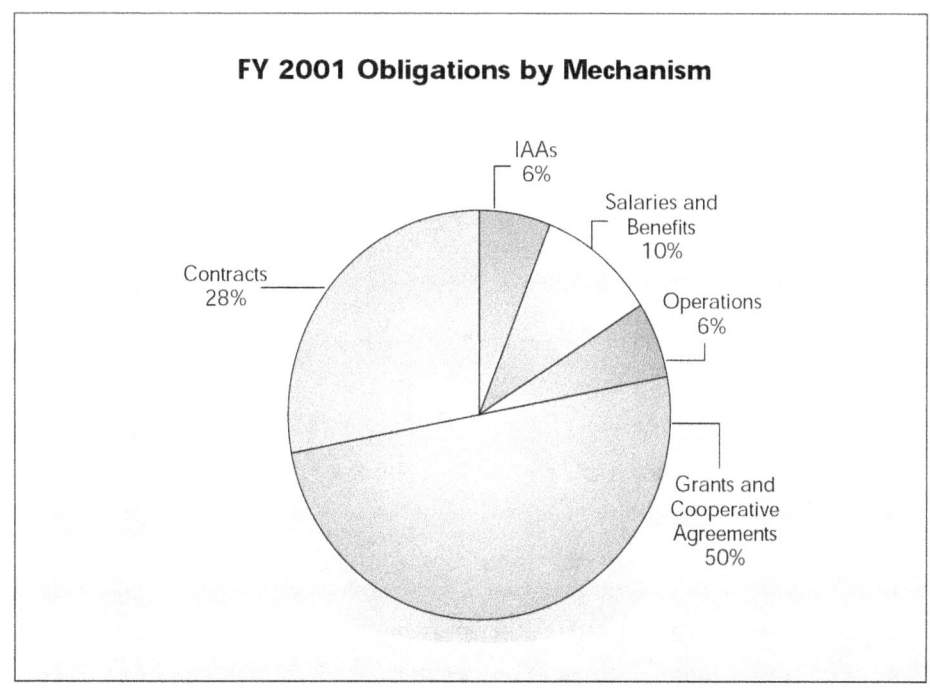

FY 2001 Obligations by Mechanism

IAAs 6%
Salaries and Benefits 10%
Operations 6%
Contracts 28%
Grants and Cooperative Agreements 50%

AHRQ uses the contract and Interagency Agreement (IAA) mechanisms to carry out a wide variety of directed health services research and administrative activities. Request for Proposals (RFPs) for contracts are announced in the Commerce Business Daily.

Analysis of Financial Statements

AHRQ's FY 2001 financial statements report the Agency's financial position and results of operations on an accrual basis. These annual financial statements are comprised of a balance sheet, statement of net costs, statement of changes in net position, statement of budgetary resources, statement of financing, and related notes that provide a clear description of the Agency and its mission as well as the significant accounting policies used to develop the statements.

Accrual Basis of Accounting	
Method of accounting that recognizes revenue when earned rather than when collected, and recognizes expenses when incurred rather than when paid.	
WHEN...	**THEN**
The order is placed.	The obligation is recorded as undelivered.
The materials are received and accepted.	The obligational authority is expended and an account payable is created.
The materials are consumed.	The material is expensed.
The Payment is made.	An outlay occurs and the account payable is cleared.

Consolidated Balance Sheet

The major components of the Consolidated Balance Sheet are assets, liabilities, and net position.

Assets

Assets represent Agency resources that have future economic benefits. AHRQ's assets totaled $287.5 million in FY 2001, an increase of close to 28 percent over the FY 2000 amount of $225.4 million. Fund balances with Treasury—mostly undisbursed cash balances from appropriated funds—comprised over 99 percent of the total assets and accounted for the entire increase over FY 2000. Fund balances represent dollars maintained at the Treasury Department to pay current liabilities, as illustrated in the accompanying graph. The increase in this category was driven primarily by the steady growth of the AHRQ appropriation over the past few years. AHRQ does not maintain any cash balances outside of the U.S. Treasury and does not have any revolving or trust funds. Less than 1 percent of AHRQ's assets were comprised of accounts receivable, which reflects funds owed to AHRQ by other Federal agencies under reimbursable agreements, funds owed to AHRQ by the public, and purchases of equipment less accumulated depreciation.

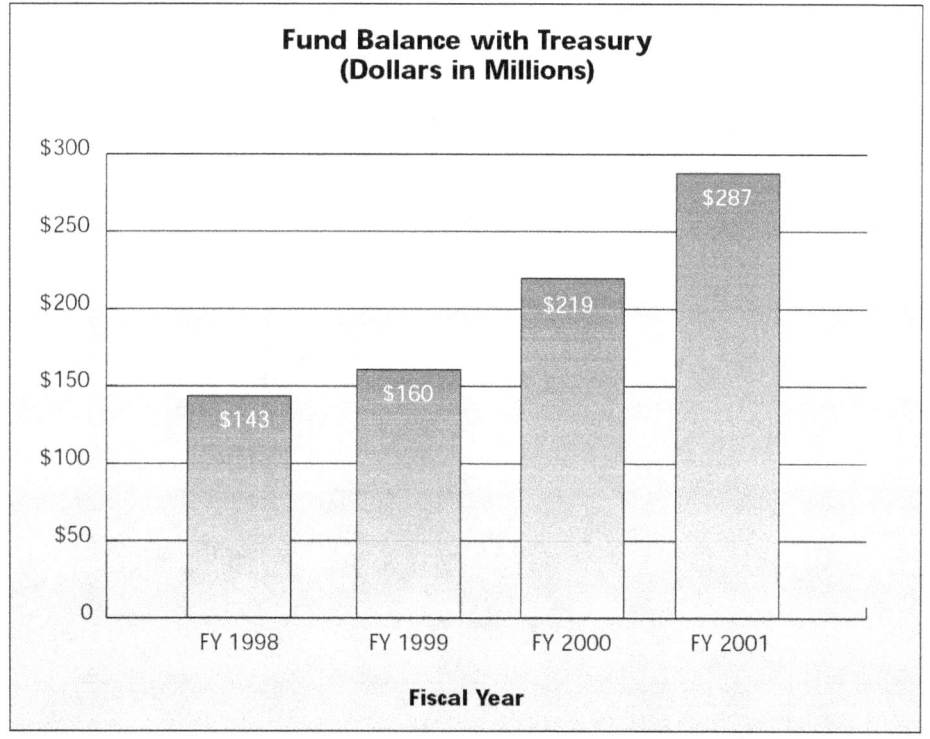

Fund Balance with Treasury
(Dollars in Millions)

Fiscal Year

Liabilities

Liabilities represent unfunded activities that require future budgetary resources. Relative to AHRQ's assets, there are few liabilities. In FY 2001, AHRQ had total liabilities of $20.7 million, an increase of $7.4 million over FY 2000. The largest components of AHRQ's liabilities were accounts payable at $11.5 million, accrued grant liabilities at $5.0 million, and accrued leave and payroll/benefit liabilities at $3.5 million. Accounts payable reflect funds owed primarily for contracts and other services. Accrued grant liabilities represent the difference between grant advances paid through the Payment Management System (PMS) and estimated grant accruals reported by the grantees. Grant advances are liquidated upon the grantee's reporting of expenditures. Accrued leave and payroll/benefit liabilities are the estimated charge for salary and funded annual and sick leave that has been earned but not paid.

71

Net Position

AHRQ's net position, which reflects the difference between assets and liabilities and signifies the Agency's financial condition, totals $266.8 million. This amount is broken into two categories: unexpended appropriations (amount of authority granted by Congress that has not been expended or used) at $89.7 million and cumulative results of operations (net results of operations since inception plus the cumulative amount of prior period adjustments) at $177.1 million. The upward change in net position was primarily the result of an increase in the funds balance with Treasury.

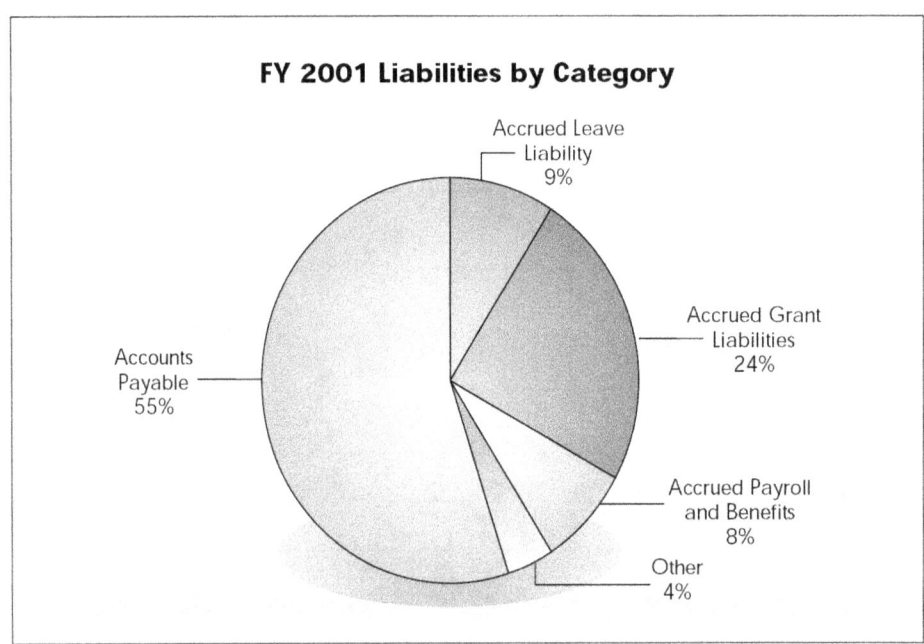

FY 2001 Liabilities by Category

Accrued Leave Liability 9%
Accrued Grant Liabilities 24%
Accounts Payable 55%
Accrued Payroll and Benefits 8%
Other 4%

Consolidated Statement of Net Cost

The Consolidated Statement of Net Cost represents the net cost to operate the Agency. Net costs, which are comprised of gross costs less earned revenues, recognize costs when incurred, regardless of the year the money was appropriated during the budget process. The categories on this statement reflect AHRQ's budget activities (major programs), thus making it possible to relate program costs to GPRA performance measures and other programs. AHRQ's FY 2001 net cost of operations was $49.1 million: $228.9 million in gross costs less $179.8 million in earned revenues.

AHRQ's net cost has decreased since FY 1999 because significant portions of AHRQ's programs were funded with PHS Evaluation Funds, which are considered earned revenues.

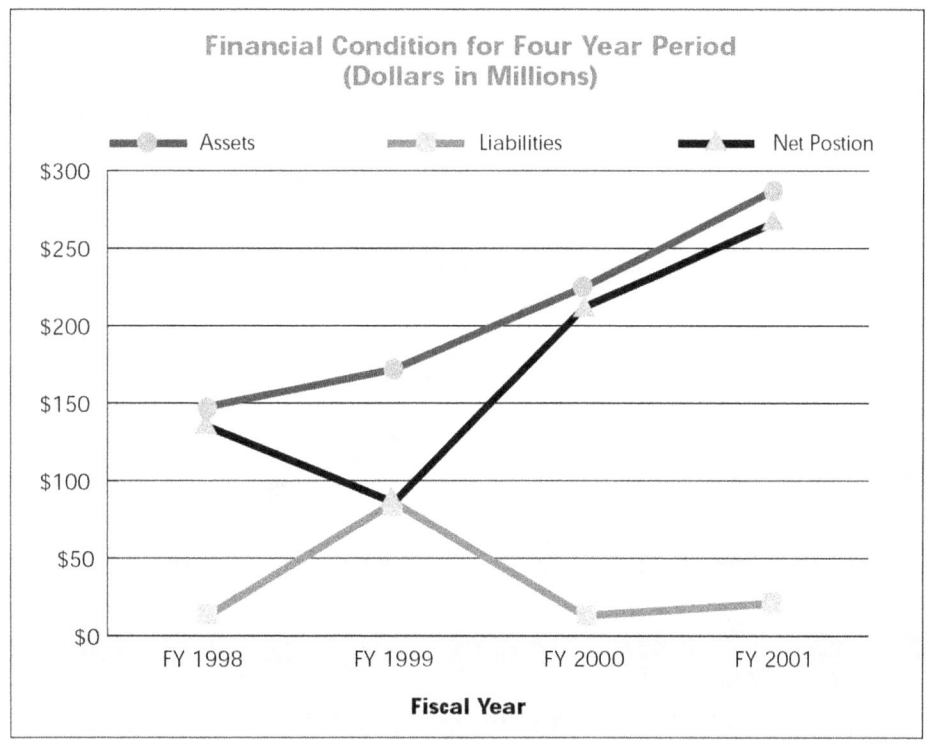

Financial Condition for Four Year Period
(Dollars in Millions)

- Assets
- Liabilities
- Net Postion

Fiscal Year

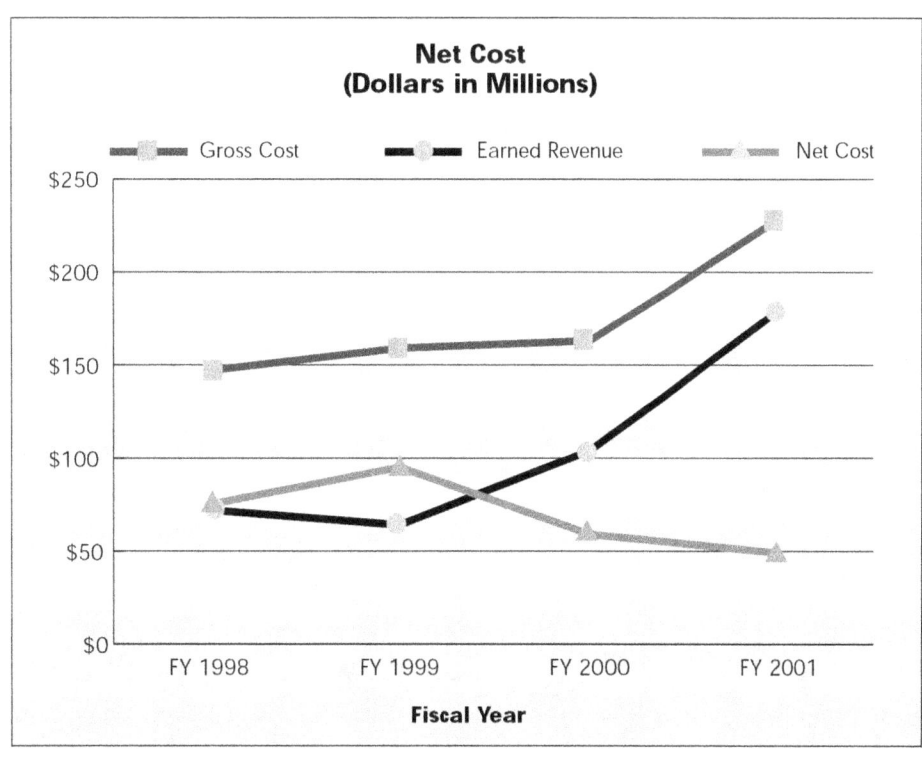

Net Cost
(Dollars in Millions)

- Gross Cost
- Earned Revenue
- Net Cost

Fiscal Year

Statement of Changes in Net Position

The Consolidated Statement of Changes in Net Position reports how the net cost of operations was financed. AHRQ ended FY 2001 with a consolidated net position total of $266.8 million, an increase of almost 26 percent from FY 2000. Net results of operations increased significantly, from $38.5 million in FY 2000 to $78.1 million in FY 2001, and appropriations used grew by $29.1 million and 30 percent. Between FY 2000 and FY 2001, unexpended appropriations decreased by $23.4 million due largely to a reduction of about $17.0 million in undelivered orders, which represent appropriations obligated but not yet received.

Statement of Budgetary Resources

The Statement of Budgetary Resources focuses on budgetary resources (appropriations and reimbursables), the status of those resources (obligated or unobligated), and the relationship between the budgetary resources and outlays (collections and disbursements). AHRQ's FY 2001 budgetary resources totaled $295.3 million and were primarily made up of spending authority from offsetting collections ($186.7 million), which includes PHS Evaluation Funds and reimbursable funds, and budget authority funds ($104.8 million). This statement shows that about 98 percent ($290.1 million) of the resources budgeted for FY 2001 were either spent or earmarked for specific activities. AHRQ's outlays

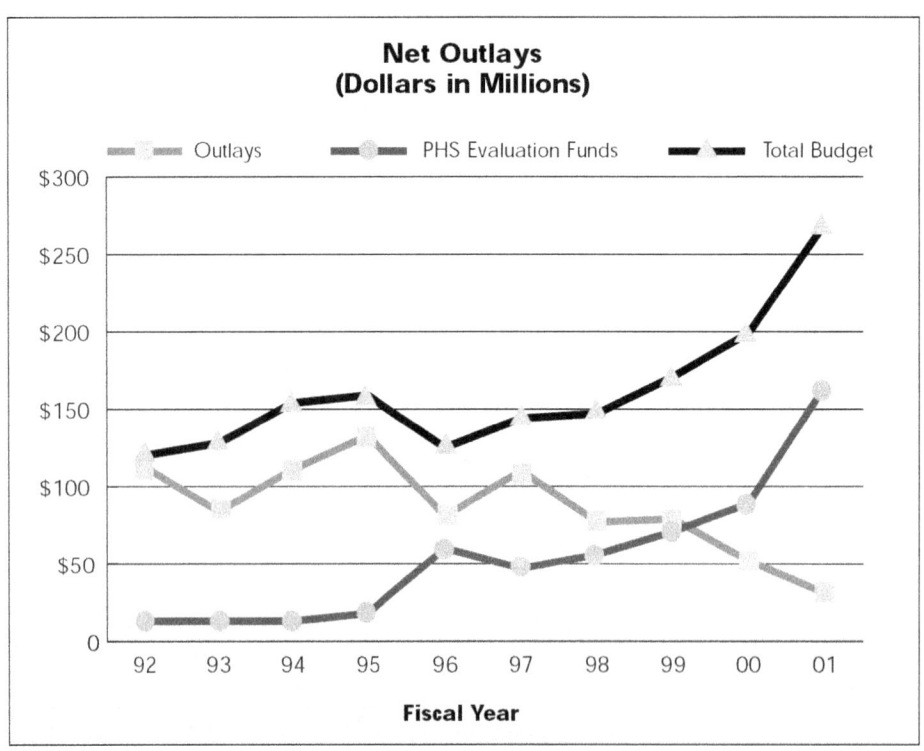

totaled $31.4 million, a decrease of 40 percent from the FY 2000 level of $52.2 million. Since 1997, the proportion of PHS Evaluation Funds to AHRQ's total budget has steadily increased, resulting in a progressive decrease of AHRQ's net outlays during the same time period.

Combined Statement of Financing

The Combined Statement of Financing links proprietary and budgetary accounting information, and reconciles obligations incurred with the net cost of operations. While the budgetary accounting system tracks resources and the status of those resources on a cash basis, the financial accounting system facilitates the translation of the use of budgetary resources into financial statements on an accrual basis. Resources that do not fund operations include changes in undelivered orders and assets purchased during the period, while costs that do not require resources include depreciation. For FY 2001, the resources used to finance AHRQ activities totaled $103.6 million, which was comprised chiefly of budgetary resources (obligations incurred less offsetting collections) as well as non-budgetary resources (costs incurred by others for AHRQ without reimbursement). The resources used to finance the net cost of operations totaled $47.5 million, while the net cost of operations totaled $49.1 million, which agrees with the amount displayed on the Consolidated Statement of Net Cost.

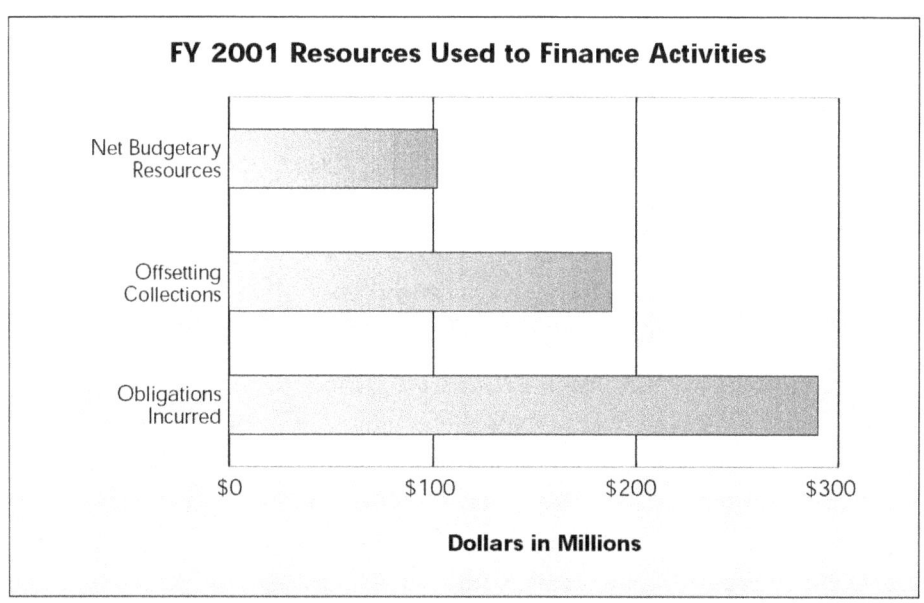

Limitations to Financial Statements

The financial statements have been prepared to report the financial position and results of operations of the entity, pursuant to the requirements of 31 U.S.C. 3515(b).

Although these statements have been prepared from the books and records of the entity in accordance with the formats prescribed by OMB, these statements are in addition to the financial reports used to monitor and control budgetary resources, which are prepared from the same books and records.

These statements should be read with the realization that they are for a component of the U.S. Government, a sovereign entity. One key implication of this fact is that liabilities cannot be liquidated without legislation that provides the resources to do so.

Other Performance Issues

Federal Managers' Financial Integrity Act (FMFIA) Efforts

The FMFIA Act of 1982 requires that Federal agencies establish processes to develop and implement appropriate, cost-effective management controls; assess the adequacy of management controls within programs and operations; identify needed improvements; and take corresponding corrective action.

In accordance with the Act, AHRQ has implemented a streamlined Management Accountability and Control Program (MAC) that uses periodic reviews, audits, and studies to provide reasonable assurance that Agency resources are protected against misappropriation, mismanagement, waste, and abuse. This Program integrates efforts to meet the requirements of FMFIA with other Agency efforts to improve effectiveness and accountability.

MAC Program activities undertaken in FY 2001 include work force planning, travel audits, IMPAC card audits, information technology security program audits, consolidation of human resource and information technology services assessments, as well as a continuing review and update of Agency operating policies and procedures. Based on an evaluation of these activities, the Agency did not identify any high-risk areas, critical weaknesses, and non-conformances in FY 2001. AHRQ also does not have any financial systems as defined by FMFIA.

The Agency remains committed to developing more efficient and effective ways to perform our mission while maintaining and protecting the integrity of the resources that have been entrusted to us. AHRQ has and will continue to use this

FY 2001 FMFIA Activities

- Completed four workforce planning related activities: evaluated the Agency's recruitment process, more clearly defined the Agency's work functions and processes, refined the technical competencies needed by Agency staff, and developed a comprehensive five-year workforce restructuring plan that reflects Agency needs and Department priorities.

- Performed periodic audits of travel documentation processed through the Travel Management System to ensure that travel expenditures conform to Department and Federal travel regulations.

- Performed periodic audits of IMPAC cardholders, focusing on the adequacy of documentation and compliance with established procedures and regulations governing card usage.

- Conducted an annual Agency-wide security program review and assessment to identify Agency information technology system and security vulnerabilities, and developed an action plan to correct all identified vulnerabilities.

- Developed and implemented a plan to consolidate the Agency's human resources staff to the Program Support Center, who in turn will provide human resource services to AHRQ under a performance based agreement.

- Institutionalized a process to allocate and when necessary, reallocate human resources to ensure that these resources are aligned with Agency strategic goals and are within budget constraints.

- Awarded a new information technology support contract using an existing National Institutes of Health resource to provide AHRQ with all Agency information technology infrastructure support as well as support for all Chief Information Officer activities including mandated security and accountability activities.

activity as an opportunity to ensure that our financial and internal management systems and controls adequately support the accomplishment of our mission.

Information Technology

Recognizing the importance of information technology (IT) for effective government, Congress enacted the Information Technology Management Reform Act (ITMRA) and the Federal Acquisition Reform Act (FAR) in 1996. These two Acts together, known as the Clinger-Cohen Act, ensure that the federal government investment in information technology is made and used wisely and introduce a set of comprehensive measures intended to improve ways that agencies acquire, use, and dispose of IT. These laws were designed to increase competition, eliminate burdensome regulations, and help the Federal government benefit from efficient private sector techniques.

Since 1996, numerous other IT-related laws established new information management requirements, including the Government Paperwork Elimination Act (GPEA) of 1998. Under GPEA, persons required to submit information to the government or maintain information must be given the option to do so electronically when practicable. That includes providing for electronic signatures and the appropriate security for the information involved. Section 508 of this Act also mandated that individuals with disabilities have access to the Federal government's electronic and information technology. This law applies to all Federal agencies when they develop, procure, maintain, or use electronic and information technology.

The Government Information Security Reform Act (GISRA), part of the 2001 Defense Authorization Act, required Federal government agencies to develop and implement comprehensive information security programs. Congress passed this law in the wake of continuing reports that Federal government systems were vulnerable to insider attacks, outside infiltration, and damage from viruses and other malicious acts. This legislation reaffirms the need for each Agency to: ensure that policies are founded on a continuous risk management cycle, implement controls that adequately assess information security risks, promote continuing awareness of information security risks, continually monitor and evaluate information security policies, and control the effectiveness of information security practices.

AHRQ also supports the Department's efforts to develop a Unified Financial Management System. This system, which will replace five existing accounting systems currently in use across the Operating Divisions, will integrate the Department's financial management structure and provide a more timely and coordinated view of critical financial management information.

AHRQ's FY 2001 accomplishments toward meeting the requirements set forth in the above laws follow.

GISRA-Related Accomplishments

- Updated and expanded AHRQ's Security Incident Response Plan.

- Reviewed AHRQ's Business Continuity and Contingency Plan.

- Performed an Agency-wide system security assessment.

- Updated AHRQ's Security Program Plan.

- Identified goals, developed action plans and preliminary implementation programs to meet GISRA objectives.

GPEA-Related Accomplishments

- Identified goals, developed action plans and preliminary implementation programs to meet GPEA objectives.

Section 508-Workforce Investment Act of 1998

- Identified goals, developed action plans and preliminary implementation programs to meet Section 508 objectives.

Financial Statements

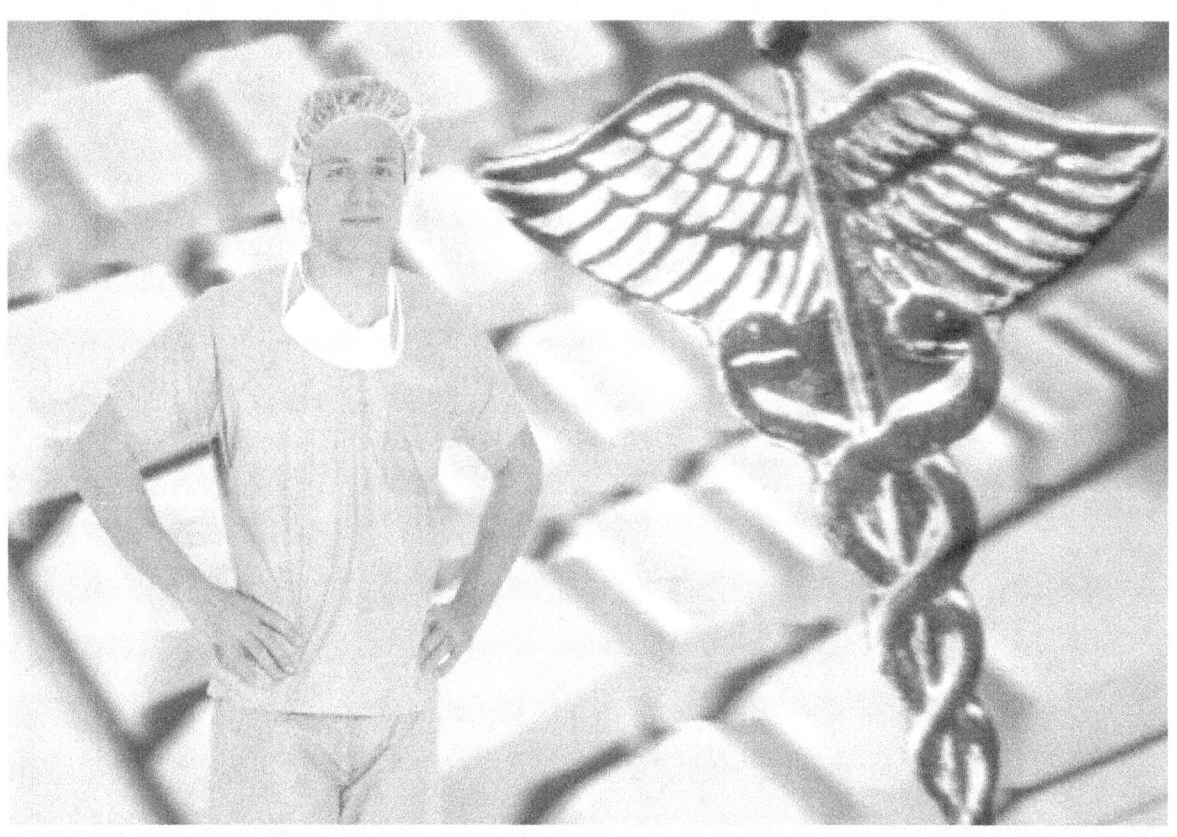

U.S. Department of Health and Human Services
Agency for Healthcare Research and Quality
CONSOLIDATED BALANCE SHEET
As of September 30, 2001 and 2000
(in thousands)

	2001	*Restated* 2000
ASSETS		
Intragovernmental		
Fund Balance with Treasury (Note 2)	$286,778	$219,029
Accounts Receivable, Net (Note 3)	1	3,763
Advances and Prepayments (Note 4)	–	40
Total Intragovernmental	286,779	222,832
Accounts Receivable, Net (Note 3)	252	48
Advances to Grantees (Note 4)	–	2,309
Advances and Prepayments (Note 4)	1	3
Property and Equipment, Net (Note 5)	435	163
TOTAL ASSETS	$287,467	$225,355
LIABILITIES		
Intragovernmental		
Accounts Payable	$1,757	$1,835
Advances from Federal Agencies		
Accrued Payroll and Benefits	311	283
Total Intragovernmental	2,068	2,118
Accounts Payable	9,706	6,357
Accrued Payroll and Benefits	1,243	1,132
Accrued Grant Liability (Note 4)	4,967	–
Actuarial FECA Liability (Note 6)	439	300
Accrued Leave Liability	1,899	3,396
Liability for Deposit Funds	328	
TOTAL LIABILITIES	20,650	13,303
NET POSITION		
Unexpended Appropriations (Note 7)	89,680	103,683
Cumulative Results of Operations	177,137	108,369
TOTAL NET POSITION	266,817	212,052
TOTAL LIABILITIES AND NET POSITION	$287,467	$225,355

The accompanying notes are an integral part of these statements.

U.S. Department of Health and Human Services
Agency for Healthcare Research and Quality
CONSOLIDATED STATEMENT OF NET COST
For the year ended September 30, 2000
(in thousands)

	Gross Cost	Less: Earned Revenues	Unaudited-Restated Net Cost
CURRENT PROGRAMS			
Research on Health Cost, Quality, and Outcomes	$135,674	$103,904	$31,770
Medical Expenditure Panel Survey	25,230	–	25,230
Program Support	2,388	–	2,388
NET COST OF OPERATIONS	$163,292	$103,904	$59,388

The accompanying notes are an integral part of these statements.

U.S. Department of Health and Human Services
Agency for Healthcare Research and Quality
CONSOLIDATED STATEMENT OF NET COST
As of September 30, 2001 and 2000
(in thousands)

	2001	Restated 2000
CURRENT PROGRAMS		
Research on Health Cost, Quality and Outcomes	$11,018	$31,770
Medical Expenditure Panel Survey	$35,555	$25,230
Program Support	2,509	2,388
Totals - Current Programs	$49,082	$59,388
NET COST OF OPERATIONS	$49,082	$59,388

The accompanying notes are an integral part of these statements.

U.S. Department of Health and Human Services
Agency for Healthcare Research and Quality
CONSOLIDATED STATEMENT OF NET COST
For the period ended September 30, 2001
(in thousands)

	Gross Cost	Less: Earned Revenues	Net Cost
CURRENT PROGRAMS			
Research on Health Cost,			
Quality, and Outcomes	$190,843	$179,825	$11,018
Medical Expenditure Panel Survey	35,555	–	35,555
Program Support	2,509	–	2,509
Total - Current Programs	$228,907	$179,825	$49,082
NET COST OF OPERATIONS	$228,907	$179,825	$49,082

The accompanying notes are an integral part of these statements.

U.S. Department of Health and Human Services
Agency for Healthcare Research and Quality
STATEMENT OF CHANGES IN NET POSITION
For periods ended September 30, 2001 and 2000

	2001	*Restated* 2000
NET COST OF OPERATIONS	$ 49,082	$ 59,388
FINANCING SOURCES (Other than exchange revenues):		
Appropriations	125,829	96,716
Donated Revenues	–	1
Imputed Financing	1,372	1,209
NET RESULTS OF OPERATIONS	78,119	38,538
PRIOR PERIOD ADJUSTMENTS	77	(29)
NET CHANGE IN CUMULATIVE RESULTS OF OPERATIONS	78,196	38,509
INCREASE (DECREASE) IN UNEXPENDED APPROPRIATIONS	(23,431)	87,856
CHANGE IN NET POSITION	54,765	126,365
NET POSITION - BEGINNING OF PERIOD	212,052	85,687
NET POSITION - END OF PERIOD	$266,817	$212,052

The accompanying notes are an integral part of these statements.

U.S. Department of Health and Human Services
Agency for Healthcare Research and Quality
STATEMENT OF BUDGETARY RESOURCES
For the year ended September 30, 2001 and 2000
(in thousands)

	September 2001	September 2000
Budgetary Resources:		
Budget Authority	$104,755	$111,402
Unobligated Balances - Beginning of Period	2,673	(493)
Spending Authority from Offsetting Collections	186,671	104,786
Adjustments	1,154	(1,240)
Total Budgetary Resources	$295,253	$214,455
Status of Budgetary Resources		
Obligations Incurred	$290,057	$212,365
Unobligated Balances - Available	1,312	815
Unobligated Balances - Not Available	3,884	1,275
Total Status of Budgetary Resources	$295,253	$214,455
Outlays		
Obligations Incurred	$290,057	$212,365
Less: Spending Authority from Offsetting Collections and Adjustments	187,825	103,546
Net Obligations Incurred	102,232	108,819
Obligated Balance, Net - Beginning of Period	218,340	161,689
Obligated Balance Transferred, Net	–	–
Less: Obligated Balance, Net - End of Period	289,128	218,340
Total Outlays	$ 31,444	$ 52,168

The accompanying notes are an integral part of these statements.

87

U.S. Department of Health and Human Services
Agency for Healthcare Research and Quality
COMBINED STATEMENT OF FINANCING
For the year ended September 30, 2001 and 2000
(in thousands)

	2001	Restated 2000
Resources Used to Finance Activities		
Budgetary		
Budgetary resources obligated for orders and delivery of goods and services to be received or benefits to be provided to others	$290,057	$212,365
Less: Offsetting collections, recoveries of prior-year authority, and changes in unfilled customer orders	187,825	103,546
Net budgetary resources used to finance activities	102,232	108,819
Non-Budgetary		
Costs incurred by others for the entity without reimbursement	1,372	1,209
Property received from others without reimbursement		
Net non-budgetary resources used to finance activities	1,372	1,209
Total resources used to finance activities	$103,604	$110,028
Relationship of Total Resources to the Net Cost of Operations:		
Increase (decr.) in budgetary resources obligated to order goods and services not yet received or benefits not yet provided	$ 56,066	$ 52,178
Total resources used to fund items not part of the net cost of operations	56,066	52,178
Resources used to finance the net cost of operations	$ 47,538	$ 57,850
Components of Net Cost of Operations that Do Not Require or Generate Resources During the Reporting Period:		
Expenses or exchange revenue related to the disposition of assets or liabilities or allocation of their costs over time:		
Expenses related to use of assets	$ 131	$ 91
Losses from re-evaluation of assets and liabilities	(272)	
Subtotal	(141)	91
Expenses that will be financed with budgetary resources recognized in future periods:		
Increase in Annual Leave Liability	335	1,253
Other	1,350	194
Total components of net cost of operations that do not require or generate resources during the reporting period	1,544	1,538
Net Cost of Operations	$ 49,082	$ 59,388

The accompanying notes are an integral part of these statements.

88

Notes to the Principal Financial Statements

Note 1 - Significant Accounting Policies

Basis of Presentation

These financial statements have been prepared to report the financial position and results of operations of the Agency for Healthcare Research and Quality (AHRQ), as required by the Chief Financial Officers Act of 1990, as amended by the Government Management Reform Act of 1994. They were prepared from AHRQ accounting records, in accordance with the form and content requirements specified by the Office of Management and Budget's (OMB) Bulletin 97-01, the Federal Accounting Standard Advisory Board's (FASAB) Statements of Federal Financial Accounting Standards (SFFASs), and AHRQ's accounting policies which are summarized in this note.

For fiscal year (FY) 2001, the Balance Sheet, Net Cost, Changes in Financial Position, Budgetary Resources, and Financing statements are repeated from prior year AHRQ reports. These statements embody the financial accounting concepts and the recognition and measurement requirements contained in the Statements of Federal Financial Accounting Concepts (SFFACs) and Standards recommended by FASAB and approved by the Secretary of the Treasury, the Director of the OMB, and the Comptroller General.

The AHRQ uses both the accrual basis and budgetary basis of accounting to record transactions. Under the accrual basis, revenues are recognized when earned and expenses are recognized when a liability is incurred, without regard to receipt or payment of cash. These financial statements were prepared following accrual accounting. Budgetary account balances are included in certain statements as appropriate. Budgetary accounting principles ensure that funds are obligated according to legal requirements. Balances on these statements therefore may differ from those on financial reports prepared pursuant to other OMB directives that are used primarily to monitor and control AHRQ's use of budgetary resources.

Reporting Entity

The AHRQ is an operating division (OPDIV) of the Department of Health and Human Services (HHS), which is a Cabinet agency of the Executive Branch of the United States Government. The AHRQ, formerly known as the Agency for

89

Health Care Policy and Research (AHCPR), was established in December 1989 under Public Law 101-239, Omnibus Budget Reconciliation Act of 1989, to enhance the quality, appropriateness, and effectiveness of health care services and access to these services. The Agency's mission is to generate and disseminate information to improve the health care system. The AHRQ is structured into the following 11 major functional components:

Office of the Director
Office of Management
Office of Priority Populations Research
Office of Research, Review, Education, and Policy
Office of Health Care Information
Center for Cost and Financing Studies
Center for Organization and Delivery Studies
Center for Outcomes and Effectiveness Research
Center for Primary Care Research
Center for Practice and Technology Assessment
Center for Quality Improvement and Patient Safety

HHS's Chief Financial Officer's (CFO) office provides the Department-wide accounting policy oversight. The Division of Financial Operations (DFO) of the Program Support Center (PSC) provides the accounting and fiscal services, including the preparation of the financial statements, on a fee-for-service basis. DFO is considered part of AHRQ's management.

The AHRQ maintains only appropriated funds. The appropriated accounts may include 1-year, multiyear, and indefinite authority. In addition, the AHRQ also uses a number of receipt, deposit, and budget clearing accounts. The financial statements report activity for the appropriated funds listed below. Also included are the related appropriation account symbols, and such activity is considered a health research and training function. AHRQ's programs are designated by OMB as falling under the health budget function category. Of AHRQ's net cost of $49.1 million, only $25.1 million was determined to be payments within the Government.

Appropriations

75X1700   Agency for Healthcare Research and Quality
75 1700   Agency for Healthcare Research and Quality

Budgets and Budgetary Accounting

Financing sources are provided through Congressional appropriations on an annual, multiyear and no-year basis, or reimbursable agreements. Annual appropriations are available for incurring obligations during a specified year; multi-year appropriations are generally available for two years. No-year or "X-year" appropriations are available for an indefinite period. For financial statement purposes, appropriations are recognized as financing sources as expenses are incurred.

Reimbursable service agreements generally recognize revenues when goods are delivered or services rendered between the AHRQ and other Federal agencies, OPDIVs, and the public. In addition, other financing sources are provided in the form of gifts from the public, interest on investments, and miscellaneous sales. All of these financing sources may be used to finance operating expenses and for capital expenditures, as specified by law.

Use of Estimates in Preparing Financial Statements

The preparation of financial statements, in conformity with generally accepted accounting principles, requires management to make estimates and assumptions. These estimates affect the reported amounts of assets and liabilities and the disclosure of contingent assets and liabilities as of the date of the financial statements, and the amounts of revenues and expenses during the reporting period. Actual results may differ from these estimates.

Fund Balances with the U.S. Treasury

AHRQ maintains all cash accounts with the U.S. Treasury. The account "Fund Balance with Treasury" represents appropriated, revolving, trust, and other funds available to pay current liabilities. The U.S. Treasury processes cash receipts and disbursements for AHRQ.

Accounts Receivable

Accounts receivable, including interest receivables, consist of amounts owed to the AHRQ by other Federal agencies and the public. The nongovernmental balances are presented net of allowances for uncollectable accounts. The allowance estimates are based on past collection experience and/or an aging analysis of the outstanding balances.

Accrued Grants

Accrued Grants are classified as non-block grants. Non-block grants draw funds to meet their immediate cash needs, and the grantees report actual disbursements (cash expenditures) quarterly. Therefore, the year-end accrual for non-block grants is equal to the estimate of the fourth quarter disbursements, plus an average of 2-week expenditures for expenses incurred without immediate cash needs.

Property, Plant, and Equipment

Property and equipment purchases and additions are valued at cost. Equipment is capitalized when cost is $25 thousand or more and it has a useful life of more than 2 years. Equipment, buildings, and capital improvements are depreciated on a straight-line basis over the estimated useful life of the asset; land is not depreciated. Routine maintenance and repair costs are expensed as incurred.

Liabilities

Liabilities are recognized for amounts of probable future outflows or other sacrifices of resources as a result of past transactions or events. Since the AHRQ is a component of the U.S. Government, a sovereign entity, its liabilities cannot be liquidated without legislation that provides resources to do so. Payment of all liabilities other than contracts can be abrogated by the sovereign entity.

Unfunded liabilities are incurred when funding has not yet been made available through Congressional appropriations or current earnings. The AHRQ recognizes such liabilities for employee annual leave earned but not taken and amounts billed by the Department of Labor (DOL) for the worker's compensation benefits. In accordance with Public Law and existing Federal accounting standards, a liability is not recorded for any future payment made on behalf of current workers contributing to the Medicare Hospital Insurance Trust Fund.

Employee Leave

Annual leave is accrued as it is earned and the accrual is reduced as leave is taken. Each year, the balance in the accrued annual leave account is adjusted to reflect current pay rates. To the extent that current or prior year funding is not available to cover annual leave earned but not taken, funding will be obtained from future financing sources. Any liability for sick leave that is accrued but not taken, funding will be obtained from future financing sources. Any liability for sick leave that is accrued but not taken by a CSRS-covered employee is transferred to the Office of Personnel Management upon the retirement of that individual. No credit is given for sick leave balances upon the retirement of FERS-covered employees.

Retirement Plans

Most AHRQ employees participate in the Civil Service Retirement System (CSRS) or the Federal Employees Retirement System (FERS). Under CSRS, AHRQ makes matching contributions equal to 7.4 percent of basic pay. Under FERS, AHRQ contributes the employer's matching share for Social Security and an amount equal to one percent of employee's pay to a savings plan. AHRQ will also match an employee's savings plan contribution up to an additional 4 percent of pay. Employees hired after December 31, 1983 are automatically covered by FERS. The Office of Personnel Management (OPM) is responsible for reporting on CSRS and FERS plan assets, accumulated plan benefits, and unfunded liabilities, if any, applicable to Federal civilian employees.

The FASAB's SFFAS Number 5, "Accounting for Liabilities of the Federal Government," requires that employing agencies recognize the full cost of pensions and health and life insurance benefits during their employees' active years of service. OPM, as the administrator of the CSRS and FERS plans, the Federal Employees Health Benefits Program and the Federal Employees Group Life Insurance Program, must provide the "cost factors" that adjust the agency contribution rate to the full cost for the applicable benefit programs. Accordingly, an imputed financing source and corresponding imputed personnel cost of $1.4 million are reflected in both the Statement of Changes in Net Position and the Statement of Net Costs, respectively. These imputed balances do not affect the AHRQ's net position.

Payroll Processing

The HHS centralized payroll system (i.e., Accounting for Pay System) computes employee payroll and benefits.

Obligations Related to Canceled Appropriations

Payments may be required of up to 1 percent of current year appropriations for valid obligations incurred against prior year appropriations that have been canceled. The total potential payments related to canceled appropriations is estimated to be $3.47 million as of September 30, 2001.

Contingencies

A contingency is an existing condition, situation, or set of circumstances involving uncertainty as to possible gain or loss to the Department/OPDIV. The uncertainty will ultimately be resolved when one or more future events occur or fail to occur. With the exception of pending, threatened, or potential litigation, a contingent liability is recognized when a past transaction or event has occurred, a

93

future outflow or other sacrifice of resources is more likely than not, and the related future outflow or sacrifice of resources is measurable. For pending, threatened, or potential litigation, a liability is recognized when a past transaction or event has occurred, a future outflow or other sacrifice of resources is likely, and the related future outflow or sacrifice of resources is measurable.

Note 2 - Fund Balances with the U.S. Treasury

AHRQ's undisbursed account balances at September 30, 2001 and 2000, are listed below by fund type. Other funds include deposit, suspense, clearing, and related non-spending accounts. AHRQ has no revolving or trust funds.

(In Thousands)	2001			2000		
	Entity Assets	Non-Entity Assets	Total	Entity Assets	Non-Entity Assets	Total
Appropriated Funds	$286,892	$ 0	$286,892	$219,069	$ 0	$219,069
Other Funds	(114)	0	(114)	(40)	0	(40)
Total	$286,778	$ 0	$286,778	$219,029	$ 0	$219,029

Note 3 - Accounts Receivable

The majority of the intra-governmental accounts receivable are the result of intra-agency and inter-agency agreements. The non-governmental accounts receivable are amounts due to the AHRQ from non-Federal sources, such as private corporations, and State and local governments.

In Thousands)	2001			2000		
	Gross Receivables	Allowance	Net Receivables	Entity Receivables	Allowance	Net Receivables
Intragovernmental	$ 1	$ 0	$ 1	$ 3,763	$ 0	$ 3,763
From the Public	1,000	(748)	252	960	(912)	48
Total	$ 1001	$ (748)	$ 253	$ 4,723	$ (912)	$ 3,811

94

Note 4 - Advances and Prepayments

Most non-governmental advances are grant advances. Other advances are emergency salary payments or travel advances.

Net Grantee Advances are paid through the Division of Payment Management's (DPM) Payment Management System (PMS). Grant advances are liquidated upon the grantee's reporting of expenditures on the quarterly PMS 272 Report, Federal Cash Transactions Report. In many cases, these reports are received several months after the grantee actually incurred the expenses reported therein. As a result, DPM and DFO estimate grant accrual amounts.

	2001	2000
Grant Advance	$ 19,838	$23,299
Less: Grant Accrual	(24,805)	(20,990)
Net Accrued Grant Advance	$(4,967)	$ 2,309

Note 5 - Property and Equipment

The AHRQ has equipment in FY 2001 with an acquisition cost of $744 thousand and accumulated depreciation of $309 thousand, with a net value of $435 thousand. In FY 2000, the acquisition cost was $341 thousand with a depreciation of $178 thousand, resulting in a net value of $163 thousand. Most buildings occupied by the AHRQ are provided by the General Services Administration (GSA). GSA charges AHRQ a Standard Level Users Charge (SLUC), which approximates commercial rental rates for similar properties. Expense for SLUC was approximately $2.6 million for FY 2001 and $2 million for FY 2000.

Note 6 - Worker's Compensation

The liability for future workers' compensation benefits includes the expected liability for death, disability, medical, and miscellaneous costs for approved compensation cases. The amount of this liability is provided to the AHRQ by the Department of Labor's Employment Standards Administration, pursuant to the Federal Employees' Compensation Act. The liability is determined using a method that uses historical benefit payment patterns, related to a specific incurred period, to predict the ultimate payment related to that period. Consistent with past

95

practice, these projected annual benefit payments (i.e., over 37 years) have been discounted to present value using the OMB's economic assumptions for 10-year Treasury notes and bonds. Interest rate assumption used for discounting for FY 2001 is 5.21 percent for year one and thereafter.

Note 7 - Unexpended Appropriations

	2001	2000
Unexpended Appropriations:		
Unobligated		
Available	$1,312	$815
Unavailable	3,884	1,275
Undelivered Orders	84,484	101593
Subtotal	89,680	103,683
Cumulative Results of Operations	177,137	108,369
Net Position	$266,817	$212,052

Note 8 - Grant Awards

The Single Audit Act of 1984, as revised, provides that recipients receiving $300 thousand or more in Federal financial assistance have an annual audit of their activities performed by an independent non-Federal auditor. The results of these audits furnish information to awarding agencies about the validity of their financial assistance award expenditures, adequacy of internal controls over Federal assistance, and the extent of compliance with grant rules and regulations. Disallowed costs identified pursuant to these audits may be used to reduce future years' grant awards, or returned to the awarding agency or general receipt funds, as required by appropriation law. Such reduction or returned awards are reported in the year the determination is made.

Final determination of allowable costs relating to grants provided by the AHRQ in FY 2000, has not been completed. Accordingly, awards issued and expensed may ultimately be adjusted for recipients' costs determined disallowed pursuant to an audit. As a result, later reviews may identify disallowances of FY 2001 expenditures after the financial statements have been issued.

Appendixes

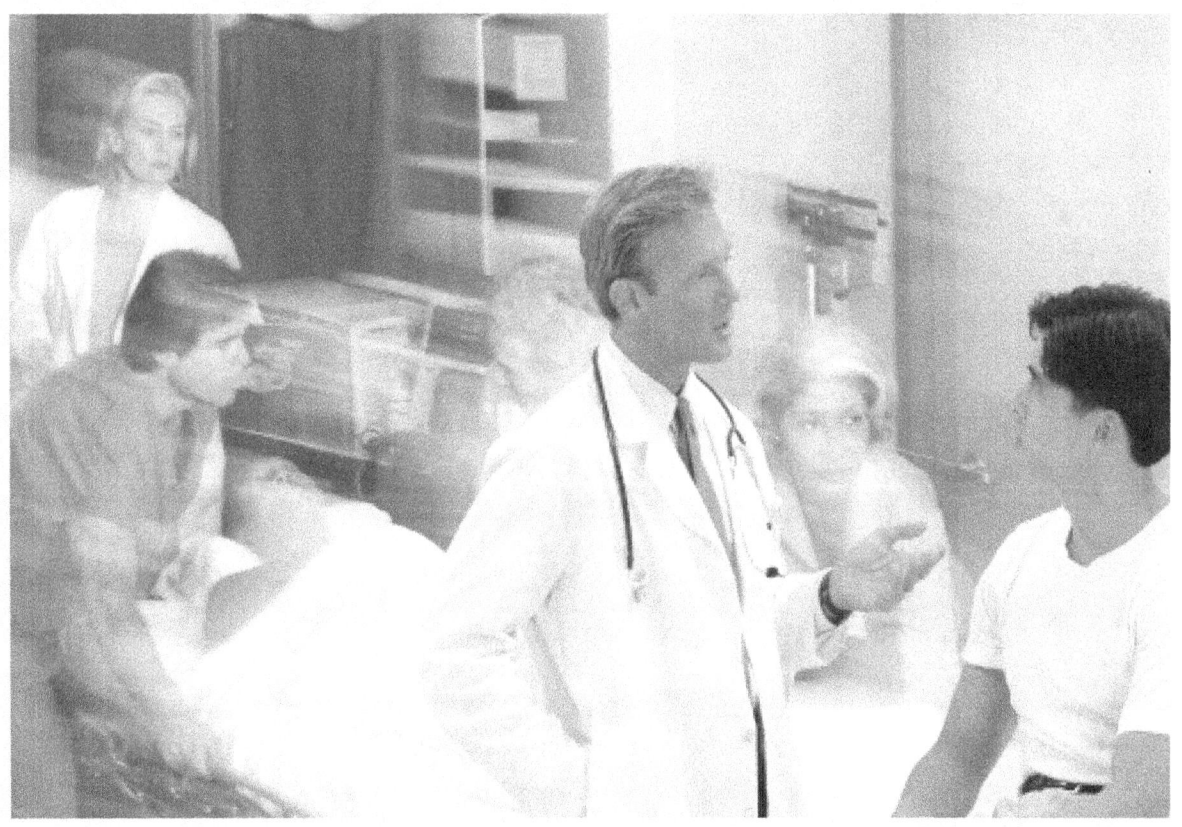

Appendix A

AHRQ's Organizational Structure

AHRQ has ten major components. They are:

- **Center for Outcomes and Effectiveness Research.** COER conducts and supports studies of the outcomes and effectiveness of diagnostic, therapeutic, and preventive health care services and procedures. Director: Carolyn M. Clancy, M.D.

- **Center for Primary Care Research.** CPCR conducts and supports studies of primary care and clinical, preventive, and public health policies and systems, including the effective application of information technology in health care. Director: Helen Burstin, M.D.

- **Center for Organization and Delivery Studies.** CODS conducts and manages studies of the structure, financing, organization, behavior, and performance of the health care system and providers within it. Director: Irene Fraser, Ph.D.

- **Center for Cost and Financing Studies.** CCFS conducts and supports studies of the cost and financing of health care and develops data sets to support policy and behavioral research and analyses. Director: Steven B. Cohen, Ph.D.

- **Center for Quality Measurement and Improvement.** CQMI conducts and supports research on the measurement and improvement of health care quality, including surveys regarding people's experiences with health care services and systems and research related to patient safety and medical errors. Director: Gregg Meyer, M.D., M.Sc.

- **Center for Practice and Technology Assessment.** CPTA directs the evidence-based practice program, consisting of: (1) the Evidence-based Practice Centers that develop evidence reports and technology assessments; (2) the Internet-based National Guideline Clearinghouse®; (3) the National Quality Measures Clearinghouse; (4) the U.S. Preventive Services Task Force; and (5) research and evaluation on translating evidence-based findings into clinical practice. CPTA also is responsible for research on the assessment of medical technologies, including conducting and sponsoring technology assessments to assist decisionmaking in other agencies. Director: Robert Graham, M.D.

- **Office of Priority Populations Research.** OPPR coordinates, supports, manages, and conducts health services research on priority populations, including racial and ethnic minorities, women, children and adolescents, the elderly, people with special needs (disabilities, chronic illness, end-of-life issues), low-income populations, and those from inner-city and rural (including frontier) areas with health care delivery issues. Acting Director: Carolyn Clancy, M.D.

- **Office of Management.** OM directs and coordinates Agency-wide administrative activities, including human resources, financial management, grant and contract management, information resources management, and other support services. Acting Director: Barry N. Flaer

- **Office of Research Review, Education, and Policy.** ORREP directs the scientific peer review process for grants and Small Business Innovation Research (SBIR) contracts, assigns projects to Agency components, plans and manages Agency health services research training and career development programs, develops and implements Agency policies and procedures regarding extramural research programs, and evaluates the scientific contribution of proposed and ongoing research, demonstrations, and evaluations. Director: Francis D. Chesley, Jr., M.D.

- **Office of Health Care Information.** OHCI designs, develops, implements, and manages programs for disseminating the results of Agency activities, including public affairs, print and electronic publishing and dissemination, reference services, research translation and synthesis, and liaison activities with State and local health policy officials. Director: Christine G. Williams, M.Ed.

Appendix B

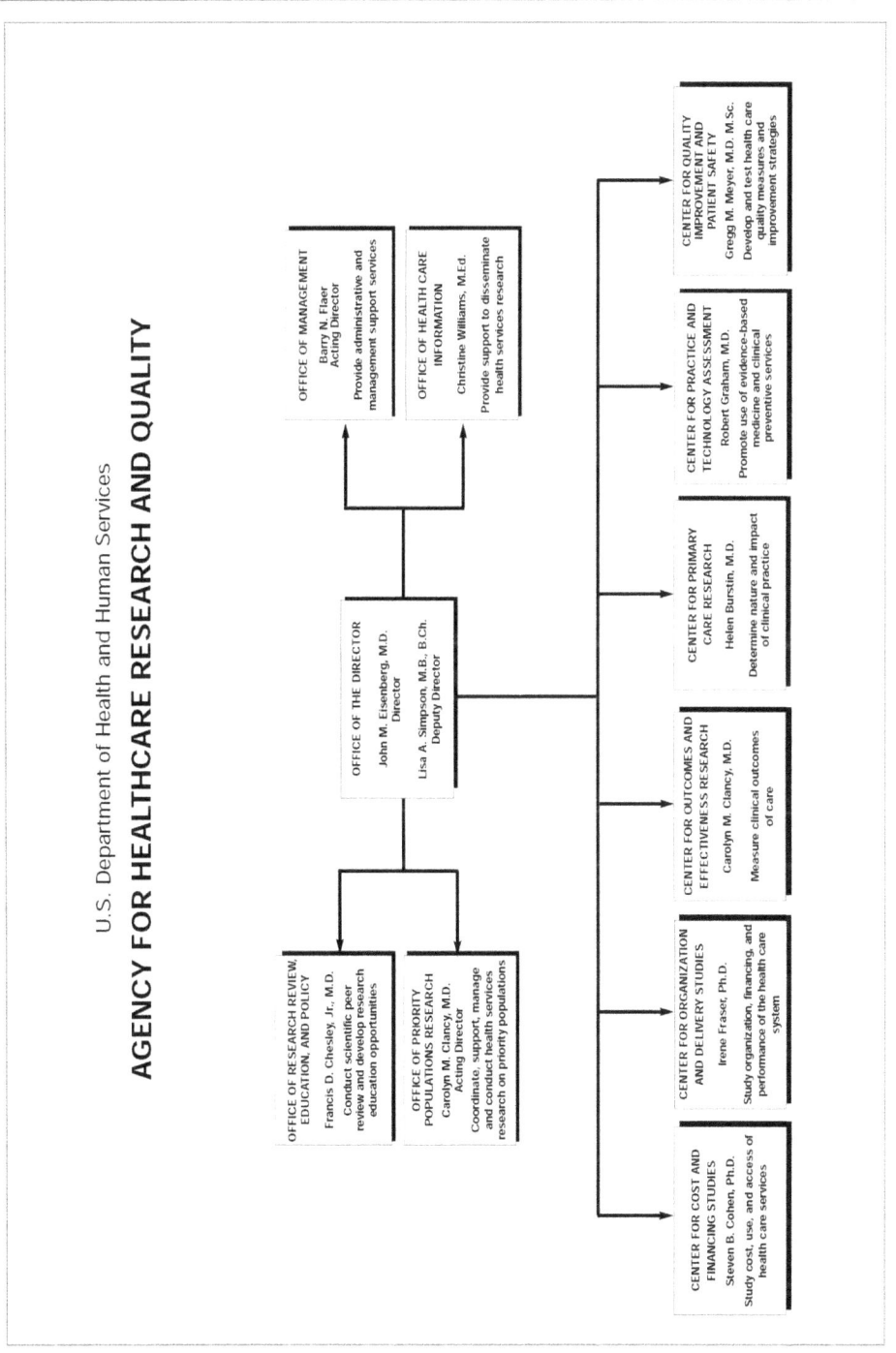

U.S. Department of Health and Human Services

AGENCY FOR HEALTHCARE RESEARCH AND QUALITY

OFFICE OF THE DIRECTOR
John M. Eisenberg, M.D.
Director

Lisa A. Simpson, M.B. B.Ch.
Deputy Director

OFFICE OF MANAGEMENT
Barry N. Flaer
Acting Director

Provide administrative and
management support services

**OFFICE OF HEALTH CARE
INFORMATION**
Christine Williams, M.Ed.

Provide support to disseminate
health services research

**OFFICE OF RESEARCH REVIEW,
EDUCATION, AND POLICY**
Francis D. Chesley, Jr., M.D.

Conduct scientific peer
review and develop research
education opportunities

**OFFICE OF PRIORITY
POPULATIONS RESEARCH**
Carolyn M. Clancy, M.D.
Acting Director

Coordinate, support, manage
and conduct health services
research on priority populations

**CENTER FOR COST AND
FINANCING STUDIES**
Steven B. Cohen, Ph.D.

Study cost, use, and access of
health care services

**CENTER FOR ORGANIZATION
AND DELIVERY STUDIES**
Irene Fraser, Ph.D.

Study organization, financing, and
performance of the health care
system

**CENTER FOR OUTCOMES AND
EFFECTIVENESS RESEARCH**
Carolyn M. Clancy, M.D.

Measure clinical outcomes
of care

**CENTER FOR PRIMARY
CARE RESEARCH**
Helen Burstin, M.D.

Determine nature and impact
of clinical practice

**CENTER FOR PRACTICE AND
TECHNOLOGY ASSESSMENT**
Robert Graham, M.D.

Promote use of evidence-based
medicine and clinical
preventive services

**CENTER FOR QUALITY
IMPROVEMENT AND
PATIENT SAFETY**
Gregg M. Meyer, M.D. M.Sc.

Develop and test health care
quality measures and
improvement strategies

Appendix C

National Advisory Council for Healthcare Research and Quality

The National Advisory Council for Healthcare Research and Quality provides advice and recommendations to AHRQ's Director and to the Secretary of the Department of Health and Human Services (HHS), on activities to enhance the quality of health care, improve health care outcomes and access to care, and reduce the costs of health care services. The 21-member council includes at least 17 private-sector experts who bring a varied perspective to the council. The private-sector members represent health care plans, clinicians, purchasers, consumers, and researchers.

Also serving as members of the council in an ex-officio capacity are the Assistant Secretary for Health, HHS, and representatives from seven Federal agencies that address health care issues: the National Institutes of Health (NIH); the Department of Defense (Health Affairs) (DoD); the Centers for Disease Control and Prevention (CDC); the Department of Veterans Affairs (VA); the Substance Abuse and Mental Health Services Administration (SAMHSA); the Food and Drug Administration (FDA); and the Centers for Medicare & Medicaid Services (formerly the Health Care Financing Administration).

The council advises the Director of AHRQ and the Secretary of HHS on:

- Priorities for health care research, especially studies related to quality, outcomes, cost, use of health care, and access to care.

- Training needs in the field of health care research and dissemination of information about health care quality.

- AHRQ's role in each of these areas in light of private-sector activity and opportunities for public-private partnerships.

Appendix D

AHRQ's Research Continuum

AHRQ's activities fall into the following three areas, which provide the steps needed to achieve the Agency's mission and goals:

1. **New research on priority health issues.** In this area, the Agency supports new research to answer important questions about what works in health care. The effort helps build the essential knowledge base to help us understand the determinants of the outcomes, quality, accessibility, and costs of care, as well as identify instances when care falls short of achieving its intended outcomes.

2. **New tools and talent for a new century.** This involves development of tools to apply the knowledge gained through the investment in new research. Here, the work of researchers is applied, and the effort begins to translate this new knowledge into instruments for measurement, databases, informatics, and other applications that can be used to assess and improve care. In addition, AHRQ provides training for the individuals who conduct this research and those who use it to build an effective and talented cadre of health services researchers and a strong research infrastructure.

3. **Translating Research into Practice.** Here is where all of the previous investment comes together. Research from the first area and the tools developed in the second area are translated into resources to close the gap between what we know and what we can do to improve health care quality. In this area, we fund research and demonstrations to translate the knowledge and tools into measurable improvements in the care Americans receive. We also develop partnerships with public- and private-sector organizations to disseminate the knowledge and tools for use throughout the health care system. This third category is a central focus of the Agency through our Translating Research Into Practice (TRIP) initiative aimed at implementing evidence-based tools and information in diverse health care settings among practitioners caring for diverse populations. The theme of translating research into practice is woven throughout all the initiatives undertaken by AHRQ in FY 2001.

AHRQ's Cycle of Research

In order to produce meaningful contributions to health care, AHRQ must set and monitor priorities, develop research initiatives based on those priorities, and keep a close watch on the processes and products that result from Agency-supported research. Four processes are involved in the AHRQ research cycle: needs assessment, knowledge creation, translation and dissemination, and evaluation.

Needs assessment. AHRQ's activities begin and finish with the end-users of our research. Our research agenda is based on an assessment of gaps in the knowledge base and the needs of patients, clinicians, health care managers, institutions, plans, purchasers, and State and Federal policymakers for evidence-based information. Needs assessment helps us shape the research initiatives undertaken by the Agency.

Knowledge creation. AHRQ continues to support and conduct research to produce the knowledge needed to improve the health care system in the coming years.

Translation and dissemination. Simply producing knowledge is not enough. Findings must be presented in ways that are useful and made widely available to clinicians, patients, health care managers, and other decisionmakers. AHRQ synthesizes and translates knowledge into products and tools that help our customers solve problems and make decisions. We are proactive in our dissemination of the knowledge, products, and tools to appropriate audiences, and we form partnerships with other organizations to leverage our resources.

Evaluation. To assess the ultimate outcomes of AHRQ research, we evaluate the impact and usefulness of Agency-supported work in health care settings and policymaking. This involves a variety of evaluation activities, including smaller, short-term projects that assess processes, outputs, and interim outcomes to larger, retrospective projects that assess the ultimate outcomes and impact of AHRQ activities on the health care system.

www.ingramcontent.com/pod-product-compliance
Lightning Source LLC
Chambersburg PA
CBHW081729170526
45167CB00009B/3751